Emergency Ultrasound

Guest Editor

JILL E. LANGER, MD

ULTRASOUND CLINICS

www.ultrasound.theclinics.com

Consulting Editor
VIKRAM S. DOGRA, MD

April 2011 • Volume 6 • Number 2

SAUNDERS an imprint of ELSEVIER, Inc.

W.B. SAUNDERS COMPANY
A Division of Elsevier Inc.

1600 John F. Kennedy Boulevard • Suite 1800 • Philadelphia, Pennsylvania 19103-2899

http://www.theclinics.com

ULTRASOUND CLINICS Volume 6, Number 2
April 2011 ISSN 1556-858X, ISBN-13: 978-1-4557-7995-6

Editor: Barton Dudlick
Developmental Editor: Donald Mumford

Ultrasound Clinics (ISSN 1556-858X) is published quarterly by W.B. Saunders, 360 Park Avenue South, New York, NY 10010-1710. Months of publication are January, April, July, and October. Business and editorial offices: 1600 John F. Kennedy Boulevard, Suite 1800, Philadelphia, Pennsylvania 19103-2899. Accounting and circulation offices: 6277 Sea Harbor Drive, Orlando, FL 32887-4800. Periodicals postage paid at New York, NY, and additional mailing offices. Subscription prices are $225 per year for (US individuals), $279 per year for (US institutions), $107 per year for (US students and residents), $253 per year for (Canadian individuals), $312 per year for (Canadian institutions), $269 per year for (international individuals), $312 per year for (international institutions), and $129 per year for (Canadian and foreign students/residents). To receive student/resident rate, orders must be accompanied by name of affiliated institution, date of term, and the signature of program/residency coordinator on institution letterhead. Orders will be billed at individual rate until proof of status is received. Foreign air speed delivery is included in all Clinics subscription prices. All prices are subject to change without notice. **POSTMASTER:** Send address changes to *Ultrasound Clinics,* Elsevier Health Sciences Division, Subscription Customer Service, 3251 Riverport Lane, Maryland Heights, MO 63043. **Customer Service (orders, claims, online, change of address): Telephone: 1-800-654-2452 (U.S. and Canada); 314-447-8871 (outside U.S. and Canada). Fax: 314-447-8029. E-mail: journalscustomerservice-usa@elsevier.com (for print support); journalsonlinesupport-usa@elsevier.com (for online support).**

Reprints: For copies of 100 or more, of articles in this publication, please contact the Commercial Reprints Department, Elsevier Inc., 360 Park Avenue South, New York, NY 10010-1710. Tel.: (+1) 212-633-3812; Fax: (+1) 212-462-1935; E-mail: reprints@elsevier.com.

Printed and bound by CPI Group (UK) Ltd, Croydon, CR0 4YY

Transferred to Digital Print 2011

Contributors

CONSULTING EDITOR

VIKRAM DOGRA, MD
Professor of Radiology, Urology, and
Biomedical Engineering, Director of Ultrasound
and Associate Chair for Education and
Research, Department of Imaging Sciences,
University of Rochester School of Medicine
and Dentistry, Rochester, New York

GUEST EDITOR

JILL E. LANGER, MD
Associate Professor of Radiology, University
of Pennsylvania School of Medicine,
Philadelphia, Pennsylvania

AUTHORS

SANDRA J. ALLISON, MD
Associate Professor of Radiology, Director,
Division of Ultrasound, Department of
Radiology, Georgetown University Hospital,
Washington, DC

MARK W. BYRNE, MD
Department of Emergency Medicine,
Brigham & Women's Hospital, Boston,
Massachusetts

KRISTIN CARMODY, MD, RDMS
Assistant Professor, Department of
Emergency Medicine, Boston University
Medical School; Director of Emergency
Ultrasound, Boston Medical Center,
Boston, Massachusetts

GHANEH FANANAPAZIR, MD
Radiology Resident, Department of
Radiology, Georgetown University Hospital,
Washington, DC

NADIM MIKE HAFEZ, MD
Clinical Instructor, Department of Emergency
Medicine, Emory University School of
Medicine, Atlanta, Georgia

MINDY M. HORROW, MD, FACR
Associate Professor of Radiology, Jefferson
Medical College, Albert Einstein Medical
Center, Philadelphia, Pennsylvania

JAMES Q. HWANG, MD, RDMS, RDCS
Harvard University, Cambridge, Massachusetts

MEGHNA KRISHNAN, MD
Clinical Fellow, Division of Diagnostic
Radiology, Abdominal Imaging Section,
Mallinckrodt Institute of Radiology,
Washington University School of Medicine,
St Louis, Missouri

SHERELLE L. LAIFER-NARIN, MD
Associate Professor of Clinical Radiology,
Director of Ultrasound and Fetal MRI,
Columbia University Medical Center,
New York Presbyterian Hospital,
New York, New York

MEGAN LEO, MD
Clinical Instructor, Department of Emergency
Medicine, Boston University Medical School;
Ultrasound Fellow, Boston Medical Center,
Boston, Massachusetts

WILLIAM MANSON, MD, RDMS, RDCS, FACEP
Assistant Professor, Director of Emergency Ultrasound, Department of Emergency Medicine, Emory University School of Medicine, Atlanta, Georgia

WILLIAM D. MIDDLETON, MD
Professor of Radiology, Division of Diagnostic Radiology, Abdominal Imaging Section, Mallinckrodt Institute of Radiology, Washington University School of Medicine, St Louis, Missouri

CHRIS MOORE, MD, RDMS, RDCS
Assistant Professor, Department of Emergency Medicine, Yale University School of Medicine, New Haven, Connecticut

SHEILA SHETH, MD, FACR
Associate Professor of Radiology and Pathology, Johns Hopkins Medical Institutions, Baltimore, Maryland

RYAN J. SMITH, MD
Clinical Assistant Professor of Radiology, Jefferson Medical College, Albert Einstein Medical Center, Philadelphia, Pennsylvania

NORA TABORI, MD
Columbia University NY Presbyterian Medical Center, PGY3 Diagnostic Radiology, New York, New York

Contents

Acute right upper quadrant pain (RUQ) is a common presentation to emergency departments. The American College of Radiology has established ultrasonography as the primary imaging tool in the evaluation of patients presenting with RUQ pain. Hence, understanding sonographic techniques and sonographic appearances of normal gallbladder, gallstones, and acute cholecystitis and their complications are pivotal in the appropriate diagnosis of patients presenting with RUQ pain. Furthermore, an understanding of the role of computed tomography, cholescintigraphy, and magnetic resonance imaging is beneficial if sonographic findings are inconclusive or require additional problem solving.

Acute pelvic pain is one of the most common symptoms prompting women to seek emergent care. The most common conditions presenting acutely include ectopic pregnancy; spontaneous abortion in pregnant women; and ovarian cysts, ovarian torsion, and pelvic inflammatory disease in nongravid patients. Despite the presence of multidetector row computed tomography in an increasing number of emergency departments, ultrasonography remains the best imaging modality for these patients. This article discusses gynecologic diseases presenting with acute or subacute pelvic pain and presents some other causes of pelvic pain that may mimic gynecologic disorders.

Up to 15% of women will experience a complication during pregnancy. Prompt diagnosis of the problem and appropriate management are imperative to a positive outcome for both the mother and the fetus. Ultrasound is the ideal imaging modality in the pregnant patient because it can be performed at the bedside, is fast, and confers no known risk to the fetus or mother. This article describes the use of ultrasound in the emergent setting. Additional correlative imaging with MRI is presented in difficult cases.

Ultrasonography is the primary imaging modality for the evaluation of acute scrotal pain and plays a critical role in differentiating between causes that require urgent surgical intervention, such as testicular torsion, and causes that can be treated medically. The ability to image the scrotal contents in real time with color and spectral Doppler, the ready availability, and the lack of ionizing radiation, make

Ultrasound may be used as an adjunct in many common procedures performed in emergency medicine, and has been demonstrated to improve effectiveness and reduce complications in diverse applications. Although the evidence is strongest for ultrasound guidance in central venous access, the use of ultrasound has been studied in many areas of procedural guidance. Emergent procedures may also be performed by consultants in a location other than the emergency department. Some of these procedures may be similar or identical to procedures performed by emergency physicians in the emergency department. This article focuses on procedures that are commonly performed by emergency physicians that may benefit from ultrasound guidance.

Ultrasound Clinics

THE CLINICS ARE NOW AVAILABLE ONLINE!

Access your subscription at:
www.theclinics.com

GOAL STATEMENT

The goal of the *Ultrasound Clinics* is to keep practicing radiologists and radiology residents up to date with current clinical practice in ultrasound by providing timely articles reviewing the state of the art in patient care.

ACCREDITATION

The *Ultrasound Clinics* is planned and implemented in accordance with the Essential Areas and Policies of the Accreditation Council for Continuing Medical Education (ACCME) through the joint sponsorship of the University of Virginia School of Medicine and Elsevier. The University of Virginia School of Medicine is accredited by the ACCME to provide continuing medical education for physicians.

The University of Virginia School of Medicine designates this educational activity for a maximum of 15 *AMA PRA Category 1 Credits*™ for each issue, 60 credits per year. Physicians should only claim credit commensurate with the extent of their participation in the activity.

The American Medical Association has determined that physicians not licensed in the US who participate in this CME activity are eligible for a maximum of 15 *AMA PRA Category 1 Credits*™ for each issue, 60 credits per year.

Credit can be earned by reading the text material, taking the CME examination online at http://www.theclinics.com/home/cme, and completing the evaluation. After taking the test, you will be required to review any and all incorrect answers. Following completion of the test and evaluation, your credit will be awarded and you may print your certificate.

FACULTY DISCLOSURE/CONFLICT OF INTEREST

The University of Virginia School of Medicine, as an ACCME accredited provider, endorses and strives to comply with the Accreditation Council for Continuing Medical Education (ACCME) Standards of Commercial Support, Commonwealth of Virginia statutes, University of Virginia policies and procedures, and associated federal and private regulations and guidelines on the need for disclosure and monitoring of proprietary and financial interests that may affect the scientific integrity and balance of content delivered in continuing medical education activities under our auspices.

The University of Virginia School of Medicine requires that all CME activities accredited through this institution be developed independently and be scientifically rigorous, balanced and objective in the presentation/discussion of its content, theories and practices.

All authors/editors participating in an accredited CME activity are expected to disclose to the readers relevant financial relationships with commercial entities occurring within the past 12 months (such as grants or research support, employee, consultant, stock holder, member of speakers bureau, etc.). The University of Virginia School of Medicine will employ appropriate mechanisms to resolve potential conflicts of interest to maintain the standards of fair and balanced education to the reader. Questions about specific strategies can be directed to the Office of Continuing Medical Education, University of Virginia School of Medicine, Charlottesville, Virginia.

The faculty and staff of the University of Virginia Office of Continuing Medical Education have no financial affiliations to disclose.

The authors/editors listed below have identified no professional or financial affiliations for themselves or their spouse/partner:

Sandra J. Allison, MD; Mark W. Byrne, MD; Kristin Carmody, MD, RDMS; Barton Dudlick, (Acquisitions Editor); Ghaneh Fananapazir, MD; Nadim Mike Hafez, MD; Mindy M. Horrow, MD, FACR; Meghna Krishnan, MD; Sherelle L. Laifer-Narin, MD; Megan Leo, MD; William Manson, MD, RDMS, RDCS; William D. Middleton, MD; Sheila Sheth, MD, FACR; Ryan J. Smith, MD; and Nora Tabori, MD.

The authors/editors listed below have identified the following professional or financial affiliations for themselves or their spouse/partner:

Matthew J. Bassignani, MD (Test Author) is on the Advisory Board/Committee for Nuance and Fuji Medical Systems.
Vikram S. Dogra, MD (Consulting Editor) is the editor for the Journal of Clinical Imaging Science.
James Q. Hwang, MD, RDMS, RDCS is on the Speakers' Bureau for 3rd Rock Ultrasound, LLC.
Jill E. Langer, MD (Guest Editor) is a consultant for Bioclinica, Inc.
Chris Moore, MD, RDMS, RDCS is a consultant for Philips Medical.

Disclosure of Discussion of Non-FDA Approved Uses for Pharmaceutical Products and/or Medical Devices.
The University of Virginia School of Medicine, as an ACCME provider, requires that all faculty presenters identify and disclose any off-label uses for pharmaceutical and medical device products. The University of Virginia School of Medicine recommends that each physician fully review all the available data on new products or procedures prior to clinical use.

TO ENROLL

To enroll in the Ultrasound Clinics Continuing Medical Education program, call customer service at 1-800-654-2452 or visit us online at www.theclinics.com/home/cme. The CME program is available to subscribers for an additional fee of $196.00.

Preface
Emergency Ultrasound

This issue of *Ultrasound Clinics* is devoted to highlighting the importance and versatility of sonography in the evaluation of patients presenting with acute symptomatology. I have asked a number of leaders in sonography from both the Radiology Community and the Emergency Department Community to share their expertise with our readers. Sonography is recognized as the primary imaging modality for the evaluation of suspected genitourinary pathology in both male and female patients, pregnancy complications, and right upper quadrant pain, and these topics are wonderfully reviewed in this issue. More recently, sonography has been effectively utilized to evaluate acute musculoskeletal injuries and acute ocular pathology. The use of focused sonography facilitates clinical decision-making and allows expedited care in patients who may not be immediately able to undergo cross-sectional imaging. The sonographic findings of a wide array of acute ocular and acute musculoskeletal conditions are beautifully illustrated. Perhaps the most unique and important feature of sonography is its real-time capabilities. The use of sonography at the bedside to assess hemodynamic physiologic changes in patients in shock and with respiratory distress is invaluable in clinical decision-making processes and allows the appropriate resuscitation of these critically ill patients. Sonography has also been demonstrated to improve effectiveness and reduce complications while performing emergent procedures such as central venous access in the critically ill. These life-saving applications of sonography are presented in this issue.

It has been an honor to serve as the guest editor. I wish to thank each author for their outstanding contribution to this issue and Barton Dudlick and his team at Elsevier for their excellent support and editorial assistance.

Jill E. Langer, MD
Department of Radiology
Hospital of the University of Pennsylvania
3400 Spruce Street
Philadelphia, PA 19104, USA

E-mail address:
jill.langer@uphs.upenn.edu

doi:10.1016/j.cult.2011.03.012

Ultrasonographic Evaluation of Right Upper Quadrant Pain in Emergency Departments

Meghna Krishnan, MD, William D. Middleton, MD*

KEYWORDS

- Right upper quadrant pain • Gallstones • Acute cholecystitis
- Ultrasound • Gallbladder disease

Acute right upper quadrant (RUQ) pain is a common reason that patients present to hospital emergency departments. The differential diagnosis is broad and most commonly encompasses disorders of the gallbladder, biliary tract, liver, subphrenic spaces, and gastrointestinal and genitourinary tracts (**Box 1**). Since the signs and symptoms of these disorders are often nonspecific and may frequently overlap, imaging is pivotal for prompt patient management.

DIFFERENTIAL DIAGNOSIS

In the emergency department setting, the primary diagnosis to be established or excluded for a patient presenting with RUQ pain is acute cholecystitis.[1–3] Acute cholecystitis, or acute inflammation of gallbladder, may develop if there is persistent cystic duct or gallbladder neck obstruction lasting more than 6 hours. In addition to pain, patients also often develop nausea, vomiting, chills, and fever. RUQ tenderness and guarding are common with acute cholecystitis. As many as 20% of patients may have mild hyperbilirubinemia,[4] and if there is common bile duct obstruction, levels greater than 4 mg per 100 ml may occur. Leukocytosis and elevations

of alkaline phosphatase, aminotransferase (transaminase), and amylase may occur.

Approximately 95% of cases of cholecystitis are because of gallstones. Gallstone disease is one of the most common medical problems leading to surgical intervention. In the United States, gallstone disease is the most common inpatient diagnosis among gastrointestinal and liver diseases.[5] The annual expenditure of $5.8 billion for gallstone treatment is exceeded only by that of gastroesophageal reflux disease.[6] Mean prevalence rates of 10% to 15% in adult Europeans and 3% to 5% in African and Asian populations have been reported.[7] In the United States, the prevalence rates range from 5% among non-Hispanic black men to 27% among Mexican-American women.[8] In American Indians, gallstone disease is epidemic and found in 73% of adult female Pima Indians.[9] In women, factors that predispose to gallstones are increased weight, increased age, and increased parity. In men, increased age also predisposes to gallstones.[10] More than 80% of gallstone carriers are unaware of their gallbladder disease.[7,11] About 1% to 2% of patients develop complications per year and often need surgery.[12] In North America, 75% of gallstones are cholesterol stones, the rest are pigment

The authors have nothing to disclose.

Division of Diagnostic Radiology, Abdominal Imaging Section, Mallinckrodt Institute of Radiology, Washington University School of Medicine, 510 South Kingshighway Boulevard, St Louis, MO 63110, USA

* Corresponding author.

E-mail address: middletonw@mir.wustl.edu

Ultrasound Clin 6 (2011) 149–161

doi:10.1016/j.cult.2011.03.004

1556-858X/11/$ – see front matter © 2011 Published by Elsevier Inc.

> **Box 1**
> **Common causes of RUQ pain**
>
> Biliary: cholelithiasis, cholecystitis, cholangitis
>
> Hepatic: abscess, hepatitis, mass, Budd-Chiari syndrome
>
> Pancreas: pancreatitis, pancreatic cancer
>
> Renal: nephrolithiasis, pyelonephritis
>
> Stomach: gastritis, peptic ulcer
>
> Bowel: appendicitis, colitis, diverticulitis, enteritis, intussusception
>
> Pulmonary: pneumonia, embolus
>
> Others: costochondritis, herpes zoster, myocardial infarction

stones.[13] Pigment stones are common in patients who have hemolytic disorders, such as sickle cell disease, biliary tract infection, or cirrhosis.

DIAGNOSTIC WORKUP OF RUQ PAIN
Nonimaging Tests

Although a careful history taking and physical examination can often provide important clues to the diagnosis of RUQ pain, the signs and symptoms of the many conditions listed in **Box 1** overlap greatly. Therefore, a number of laboratory tests are relatively routine. Liver function tests are helpful because certain abnormalities can strongly suggest hepatobiliary disease, and the pattern of abnormality on these tests can point toward liver parenchymal processes or biliary processes. Renal, pancreatic, and cardiac abnormalities can be identified in many cases by obtaining a urinalysis, serum amylase and lipase levels, and an electrocardiograph, respectively.

An evidence-based diagnosis of acute cholecystitis was studied in a meta-analysis published in 2003,[14] which showed that no clinical or laboratory finding had a high or low enough likelihood ratio to predict the presence or absence of acute cholecystitis. This study further supported the evidence that imaging studies are essential for establishing or excluding the diagnosis of acute cholecystitis and for the establishment or exclusion of alternate diagnoses, if acute cholecystitis is not present.

Imaging Tests

A wide variety of imaging techniques exist to evaluate patients with RUQ pain. These techniques include chest and abdominal radiography, luminal studies of the gastrointestinal tract, ultrasonography (US), biliary scintigraphy, computed tomography (CT), and magnetic resonance (MRI).

The American College of Radiology revised the appropriateness criteria for imaging tests for evaluating patients presenting with RUQ pain in 2010.[15] A rating scale of 1 (usually not appropriate) to 9 (usually appropriate) is used to denote relative appropriateness of imaging tests that are used for evaluating patients presenting with RUQ pain. In addition to RUQ pain, if a patient has clinical findings of fever, elevated white blood cell count, and a positive clinically elicited Murphy sign, then the primary imaging test recommended with the highest rating of 9 is US. Abdominal CT (preferably with contrast), cholescintigraphy, and abdominal MRI with or without contrast each have a rating of 6 and should be performed only if sonographic findings are inconclusive or require additional problem solving. Even if the patient presents with RUQ pain without fever, elevated white blood cell count, or Murphy sign, the imaging test of choice with a rating of 9 remains US. CT, cholescintigraphy, and MRI, each with a rating of 6, are recommended only if sonographic findings are inconclusive or require additional problem solving. Abdominal US has been rated 9 in most variants of clinical presentation of patients with RUQ pain, except in acalculous cholecystitis in which it is rated 8. Even in that setting for acalculous cholecystitis, the other imaging modalities are rated only 6 or less.

Some of the reasons for which US is the preferred imaging test in patients with RUQ pain include better availability, lack of ionizing radiation, better morphologic evaluation of the gallbladder for complications, confirmation of the presence or absence of gallstones, evaluation of intrahepatic and extrahepatic bile ducts, and identification or exclusion of alternative diagnoses.[1,16–18] The positive predictive value of sonography in identifying patients who would benefit from cholecystectomy is 99%.[19]

When sonographic evaluation is nonconclusive for acute cholecystitis, scintigraphy is often the next imaging test of choice. Cholescintigraphy has been reported to have similar accuracy for the diagnosis of acute cholecystitis.[20] Several investigations have directly compared the accuracy of cholescintigraphy and US for the diagnosis of acute cholecystitis.[21] These studies have shown an overall sensitivity and specificity of 86% to 97% and 73% to 100%, respectively, for cholescintigraphy and 81% to 100% and 60% to 100%, respectively, for US.[22–25] However, scintigraphy is incapable of diagnosing nonbiliary conditions and up to two-thirds of patients seen in the emergency department with suspected cholecystitis do not have cholecystitis. In addition, the longer time required to perform scintigraphy (up to 4 hours to separate acute from chronic cholecystitis) is a limitation. This time can, however, be diminished by half, with the use of intravenous morphine. If the sonogram is confusing or inconclusive, scintigraphy should be considered as a powerful problem solver, provided it would potentially change patient management.[25]

Abdominal CT can be valuable when US results shows a complex process centered over the gallbladder, and the differential diagnosis includes both complicated cholecystitis and gallbladder cancer. Abdominal CT is also needed in some cases to distinguish emphysematous cholecystitis from porcelain gallbladder (see later). In addition, when sonography shows a normal stone-free gallbladder and no other explanation for the patient's pain, then CT can be very helpful to survey the entire abdomen to identify alternative diagnoses. MRI/magnetic resonance cholangiopancreatography examination is generally obtained to better characterize masses in the liver or other solid organs identified on US or to search for possible obstructive process in the extrahepatic biliary tree. This technique is especially applicable when the US examination was technically challenging to perform because of the patient's body habitus or when extensive bowel gas compromises the sonographic examination.

NORMAL GALLBLADDER

The normal gallbladder is a fluid-filled ovoid structure with a thin, smooth echogenic wall (**Fig. 1**). The gallbladder is located inferior to the interlobar fissure between the left and right hepatic lobes.

Anatomically, the gallbladder is divided into the neck, body, and fundus. The neck of the gallbladder generally lies closest to the liver hilum. Folds in the gallbladder commonly occur at the neck and fundus. The spiral valves of Heister are small folds in the cystic duct or gallbladder neck; they can appear as tiny protuberances in the cystic duct and should not be confused for stones or polyps (**Fig. 2**). The fundus is variable in position and can be located anywhere from the diaphragm to the iliac crest.

The gallbladder wall normally has a thickness less than 3 mm in a fasted patient. The wall can appear thickened if the gallbladder is contracted, but even in the contracted state, the wall thickness usually does not exceed 3 mm (**Fig. 3**). The transverse (short axis) diameter of the gallbladder should be shorter than 4 cm. The gallbladder length is more variable and less useful diagnostically, but a reasonable upper limit of normal length is 8 to 10 cm.

TECHNIQUE

Ideally, patients should fast for 6 to 8 hours for a gallbladder sonogram to ensure adequate gallbladder distension and to reduce upper abdominal bowel gas. Fasting prevents contraction of the gallbladder and allows for better detection of stones and better evaluation of the wall. However, fasting may not be always feasible in a patient presenting to the emergency department with acute RUQ pain, and a recent meal is not a contraindication to sonography in this situation.

A midfrequency (3–5 MHz) sector transducer is typically used to scan the gallbladder and right upper abdomen. In unusually thin patients, higher-frequency linear or curved arrays can be used to obtain higher-resolution images. In unusually

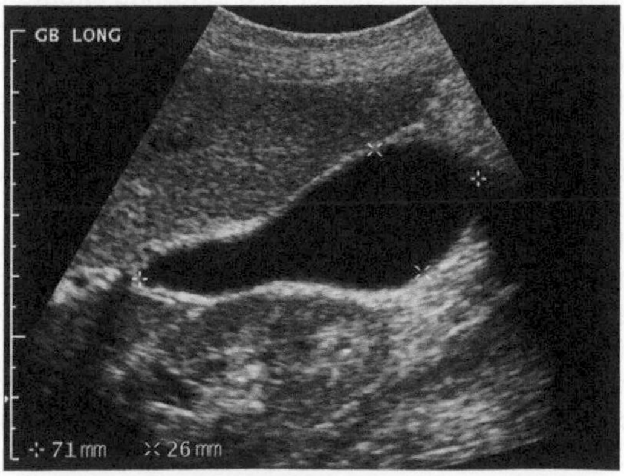

Fig. 1. Normal gallbladder. Longitudinal view shows an oval-shaped gallbladder with a thin wall measuring 7.1 × 2.6 cm.

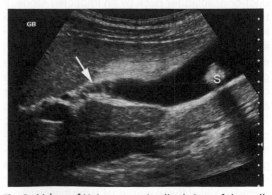

Fig. 2. Valves of Heister. Longitudinal view of the gallbladder neck shows small closely spaced folds at the origin of the cystic duct (*arrow*). A stone (S) is also present in the body of the gallbladder.

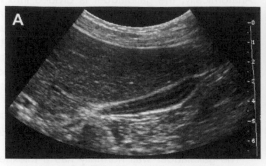
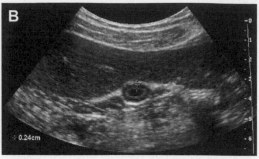

Fig. 3. Contracted gallbladder. (*A*) Longitudinal view shows a very narrow lumen measuring approximately 5 mm. Note the apparent wall thickening. (*B*) Transverse view shows that despite the appearance of wall thickening, the wall is within normal limits measuring only 2.4 mm.

obese patients, lower-frequency phased-array transducers may be necessary. Harmonic imaging and real-time compounding are helpful for both eliminating artifactual echoes and accentuating real echoes from the gallbladder, especially in obese patients.

The gallbladder is usually best seen from a subcostal approach with the patient in a left lateral decubitus or left posterior oblique position during deep inspiration. If the gallbladder is unusually high, an intercostal window may be necessary. Imaging should be performed with the patient in prone and upright positions to help visualize stones that might otherwise be hidden in the gallbladder neck and to assess for mobility of any detected stones. Careful attention should be paid to both the neck and fundus of the gallbladder because stones can sometimes hide in these locations.

Acute Cholecystitis

In most patients, acute cholecystitis occurs because of persistent obstruction of the cystic duct or gallbladder neck by an impacted stone. If the obstructing process is not removed or if the inflammation of gallbladder continues, necrosis and perforation of the gallbladder wall may occur, eventually leading to peritonitis and sepsis. Sonographic findings that favor a diagnosis of acute cholecystitis include (1) gallstones, (2) gallbladder enlargement, (3) gallbladder wall thickening, (4) impacted stone in the gallbladder neck or cystic duct, (5) pericholecystic fluid, and (6) focal tenderness directly over the gallbladder (positive sonographic Murphy sign). A combination of these signs in the appropriate clinical setting is important because any of these individual signs in isolation is nonspecific. For instance, gallstones are generally required to make the diagnosis of cholecystitis, but most patients with stones detected on

sonography do not have cholecystitis. However, the combination of gallstones and a positive sonographic Murphy sign has a positive predictive value of 92% and a negative predictive value of 95%.[19] Additional sonographic findings in more advanced acute cholecystitis include (1) sloughed mucosal membranes, (2) wall disruption, (3) wall ulceration, and (4) focal bulge of the wall.

Gallstones

Approximately 95% of patients with acute cholecystitis have gallstones. So, detection of stones is an extremely important aspect for the evaluation of acute cholecystitis. Sonography has a sensitivity of greater than 95% for detecting stones. This test is more sensitive than any other test, and therefore, sonography has assumed the primary role in the evaluation of suspected acute cholecystitis. In addition, the negative predictive value of sonography for gallstones is greater than 97%, so sonography is very accurate in excluding cholecystitis by showing a stone-free gallbladder.

The typical sonographic appearance of a gallstone is a mobile, echogenic, shadowing structure in the lumen of the gallbladder (**Fig. 4**). Shadowing and mobility are important because they help distinguish stones from masses and tumefactive sludge. Shadowing is primarily related to stone size and not to stone composition. For shadow production, the ultrasound beam should intercept the center of the stone and the stone should absorb a critical portion of the sound pulse, which is rarely a problem when stones are large in relation to the beam width. With small stones, however, adjusting the focal zone of the beam to correspond to the depth of the stone is critical. Using a higher-frequency transducer (**Fig. 5**) and inactivating the compound imaging feature (**Fig. 6**) also improve the chances of demonstrating shadowing with small stones. If shadowing is not

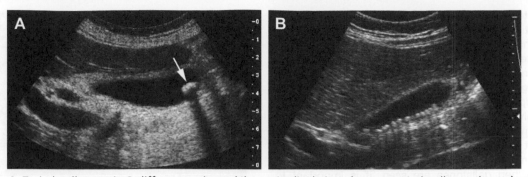

Fig. 4. Typical gallstones in 2 different patients. (*A*) Longitudinal view shows a typical gallstone (*arrow*) with a strong acoustic shadow. (*B*) Longitudinal view shows multiple smaller stones with weak acoustic shadows.

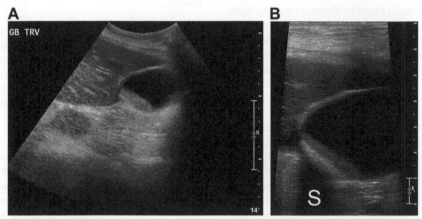

Fig. 5. Effect of transmit frequency on shadowing. (*A*) Transverse view obtained with a 5-MHz curved array probe shows echogenic nonshadowing material in the dependent portion of the gallbladder. (*B*) Similar view with a 9-MHz linear array probe shows shadowing. The presence of shadowing changes the diagnosis from sludge to a combination of sludge and small stones (S).

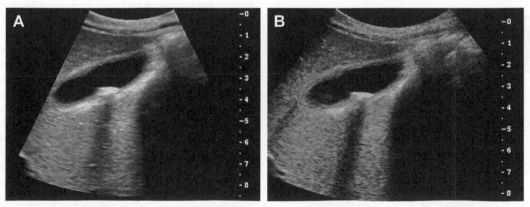

Fig. 6. Effect of real-time compounding on shadowing. (*A*) Longitudinal view obtained with active compounding shows stones with a faint shadow. (*B*) Similar view with inactive compounding shows a much stronger shadow.

detected despite all these adjustments, the differential includes gallstones and tumefactive sludge. Small, mobile, nonshadowing, intraluminal structures are generally gallstones. Tumefactive sludge generally forms larger masslike aggregates (**Fig. 7**). Occasionally, a follow-up sonogram is helpful to distinguish between these 2 possibilities. Polyps and other masses may also simulate small nonshadowing stones, but unlike stones, they are not mobile and are not necessarily in the dependent portion of the gallbladder (**Fig. 8**).

When gallstones are seen, it is important to determine if they are mobile when changing the patient's position: turning the patient to the left or right or to a prone or upright position may cause the gallstone to move to a dependent position (**Fig. 9**). Occasionally, if gallstones are numerous, they may not appear to be mobile because there may not be enough room to move. In some cases, it is possible to identify the impacted stone that is causing the obstruction in the gallbladder neck (**Fig. 10**). However, it is not unusual to see mobile nonobstructing stones in the lumen without visualization of the obstructing stone in the cystic duct.

Occasionally, when the gallbladder is filled with a large stone or an aggregate of multiple stones, it produces a wall-echo-shadow complex (**Fig. 11**). The presence of this complex often indicates a contracted and diseased gallbladder that is unable to perform its primary function of storing bile, but it is rarely seen with acute cholecystitis. This sign comprises 3 arc-shaped lines.[26] The gallbladder wall appears as a central hypoechoic line. Deep to this line, an echogenic line arises from the stones. Deeper to this echogenic line is the intense dark acoustic shadowing. Also seen is an echogenic line representing pericholecystic fat at the interface of the gallbladder wall and liver.

When the specific gravity of bile is unusually high and exceeds the specific gravity of stones, the stones may float. This lower specific gravity

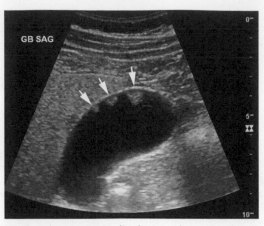

Fig. 8. Polyps. Longitudinal view shows 3 adjacent echogenic lesions on the nondependent wall of the gallbladder (*arrows*). None of these structures were mobile.

indicates that the floating stones are composed of cholesterol. These floating stones are most frequently seen after intravenous injection of iodinated contrast when there has been vicarious excretion of contrast into the gallbladder. The presence of floating stones has no particular association with acute cholecystitis.

Gallbladder Wall Thickening

Gallbladder wall thickening greater than or equal to 3 mm is present in many patients with acute cholecystitis (**Fig. 12**). The positive predictive value of the combination of gallstones and wall thickening (in a population of patients with a prevalence of cholecystitis of 62%) is 94%. The negative predictive value of this combination is 98%.[19]

It is important to realize that in most cases of acute cholecystitis, the wall thickening is not severe. It is also important to remember that there are many other causes of wall thickening, which are listed in **Box 2**. The gallbladder wall is particularly prone to edema and can become visibly thickened because of a large variety of causes other than cholecystitis. Therefore, conditions causing systemic edema, such as heart failure, renal failure, and hypoproteinemia, are very common causes of gallbladder wall thickening. Adjacent inflammatory processes such as hepatitis and pancreatitis are also relatively common. Conditions that effect venous outflow from the liver and gallbladder, such as cirrhosis, portal hypertension, and portal vein thrombosis, are also causes of gallbladder wall thickening. One common misconception is that ascites is a cause of gallbladder wall thickening. It is true that ascites and wall thickening frequently coexist, but there is no cause-and-effect relationship. The nonbiliary

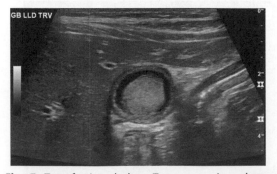

Fig. 7. Tumefactive sludge. Transverse view shows a round nonshadowing structure in the gallbladder lumen. Doppler views showed no detectable internal vascularity.

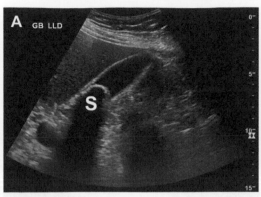
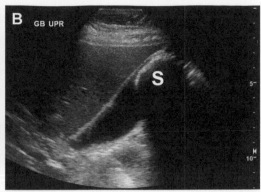

Fig. 9. Gallstone mobility. (*A*) Longitudinal view of the gallbladder with the patient in a left lateral decubitus shows a large stone (S) in the gallbladder neck. (*B*) Similar view with the patient in an upright position shows that the stone (S) has moved into the fundus, thus excluding the possibility of stone impaction.

causes of wall thickening typically produce the most markedly thickened walls that one will encounter and walls that are thicker than typically seen with acute cholecystitis. Therefore, a thick gallbladder wall in the absence of stones, gallbladder enlargement, or a positive Murphy sign should certainly not be equated with cholecystitis, and a careful survey for sonographic signs of heart failure, cirrhosis, pancreatitis, or other nonbiliary causes of wall thickening should be performed (**Fig. 13**). Patients with asymptomatic nonimpacted gallstones and wall edema from nonbiliary causes can be a diagnostic challenge sonographically. In the proper clinical setting,

scintigraphy can be very helpful in further evaluating this type of patient.

Adenomyomatosis is another cause of gallbladder wall thickening that can potentially be confused with acute cholecystitis. The focal and segmental forms of adenomyomatosis rarely simulate cholecystitis, but the diffuse form can occasionally pose diagnostic problems. In most cases, the clinical history is very helpful because adenomyomatosis is largely asymptomatic. Useful sonographic signs are intramural comet tail artifacts that arise from crystals within Rokitansky-Aschoff sinuses, as well as a lack of gallbladder enlargement and a negative Murphy sign (**Fig. 14**).[27] Although rarely needed, an MRI can sometimes identify Rokitansky-Aschoff sinuses that are sonographically occult and assist in the diagnosis of adenomyomatosis.

Fig. 10. Acute cholecystitis with an impacted stone. Longitudinal view of the gallbladder shows several stones in the lumen. An additional stone that was originally overlooked is impacted at the junction of the neck and the cystic duct (*arrow*). (*Data from* Middleton W, Kurtz A. Ultrasound: the requisites. 2nd edition. Philadelphia: Mosby; 2004. p. 37.)

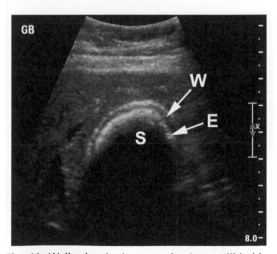

Fig. 11. Wall-echo-shadow complex in a gallbladder completely filled with stones. Transverse view of the gallbladder shows the hypoechoic wall (W), the echogenic reflection from the stones (E), and the shadow (S).

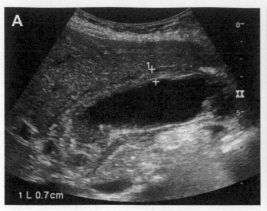
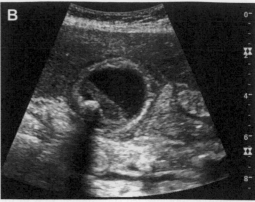

Fig. 12. Acute cholecystitis with gallbladder wall thickening. (*A*) Longitudinal view of the gallbladder shows a thickened wall measuring 7 mm. (*B*) Transverse view also shows a thick wall in addition to a stone and sludge.

It has been reported that the sensitivity and specificity of diagnosing acute cholecystitis can be improved with color and power Doppler US evaluation of the gallbladder wall.[28] However, in most situations, Doppler evaluation is not necessary and adds little to the diagnosis.

Gallbladder Enlargement

Gallbladder enlargement is an additional sign of acute cholecystitis. In the appropriate clinical setting, an enlarged gallbladder should raise suspicion of acute cholecystitis, and a careful

---

Box 2
Differential diagnosis of thickened gallbladder wall

- Physiology

  o Contraction of the gallbladder because of the recent consumption of a fatty meal

- Gallbladder disease

  o Acute cholecystitis
  o Acute acalculous cholecystitis
  o Adenomyosis
  o Gallbladder cancer

- Nongallbladder disease

  o Cirrhosis/portal hypertension
  o Portal vein thrombosis
  o Pancreatitis
  o Acute hepatitis
  o Hypoproteinemia
  o Congestive cardiac failure
  o Renal failure

Data from Chong W, Shah M. Sonography of right upper quadrant pain. Ultrasound Clin 2008;3(1):122.

---

search for additional signs should be performed (**Fig. 15**). However, like most signs of cholecystitis, gallbladder enlargement by itself is neither highly sensitive nor highly specific. As mentioned earlier, a normal gallbladder generally has a width less than 4 cm and a length less than 8 to 10 cm. The width is a more important dimension because of the normal variation in gallbladder length. A long thin gallbladder is much less worrisome than a short wide gallbladder.

Pericholecystic Fluid

Pericholecystic fluid is present in less than 20% of patients with acute cholecystitis. It is seen as a focal fluid collection adjacent to the gallbladder wall (**Fig. 16**). Pericholecystic fluid can appear anywhere around the circumference of the gallbladder but is most often adjacent to the fundus. Recognizing this fluid is important because it generally indicates a more advanced case of cholecystitis. Pericholecystic fluid should be differentiated from gallbladder wall edema, which is more concentric. Pericholecystic fluid should also be distinguished from pericholecystic ascites, which is less masslike and conforms to the shape of the gallbladder and adjacent structures.

Sonographic Murphy Sign

The sonographic Murphy sign refers to localized tenderness directly over the gallbladder. This sign is considered positive when pressure applied with transducer elicits tenderness only over the gallbladder or when maximal tenderness is located over the gallbladder. As mentioned earlier, a combination of gallstones and a positive sonographic Murphy sign has a positive predictive value of 92%.[19] A negative sonographic Murphy sign is less helpful. Causes of a false-negative

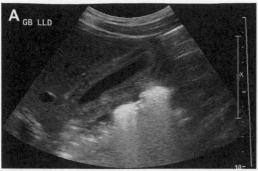
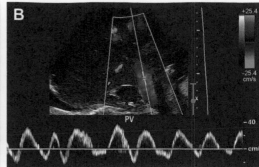

Fig. 13. Heart failure with gallbladder wall thickening. (*A*) Longitudinal view of the gallbladder shows diffuse concentric wall thickening, but no stones, and a somewhat contracted lumen. (*B*) Pulsed Doppler waveform from the portal vein shows abnormal pulsatility consistent with congestive heart failure and passive hepatic congestion.

Murphy sign include patient nonresponsiveness, pain medication, diabetic patient, or inability to press directly on the gallbladder because of large ascites or deeply positioned gallbladder either deep to liver or ribs. A very important cause of a negative Murphy sign is gallbladder wall necrosis, which leads to denervation of the gallbladder wall by gangrenous changes.

Acalculous Cholecystitis

Acute acalculous cholecystitis accounts for approximately 5% of all cases of acute cholecystitis and occurs most commonly in patients in intensive care units. Predisposing factors include trauma, mechanical ventilation, hyperalimentation, postoperative state, diabetes mellitus, vascular insufficiency, prolonged fasting, burns, and postpartum state. These conditions tend to increase the risk for gallbladder ischemia. Patients with suspected acalculous cholecystitis are challenging to assess clinically, and an increased morbidity and mortality rate are partly because of the difficulty

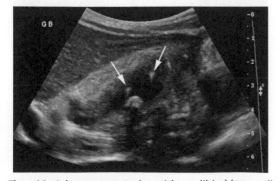

Fig. 14. Adenomyomatosis with gallbladder wall thickening. Longitudinal view of the gallbladder shows a thick wall, a gallstone, and several intramural reflectors with comet tail artifacts (*arrows*).

and delay in making the diagnosis. The sonographic features of enlargement and wall thickening that are useful in other populations of patients are also signs of acalculous cholecystitis (**Fig. 17**). However, these features frequently exist in patients in the intensive care unit without intrinsic gallbladder disease. Therefore, the sonographic evaluation of these patients is also difficult. Scintigraphy can be a helpful adjunct to sonography, but false-positives are common and limit its usefulness. As a result, guided cholecystostomy tube placement is often performed to decompress the gallbladder if there is a high index of clinical suspicion and the gallbladder is distended on US results.[29]

Gangrenous Cholecystitis

Increased intraluminal pressure in the gallbladder from acute cholecystitis may produce gallbladder wall ischemia and ultimately necrosis, resulting in gangrenous cholecystitis. Gangrenous cholecystitis complicates 2% to 38% of cases.[30] The sonographic Murphy sign may be negative in a large number of these patients, probably because of denervation of the gallbladder wall by gangrenous changes.[31] Progression of gangrenous cholecystitis can lead to perforation of gallbladder, resulting in peritonitis and sepsis, leading to higher morbidity and mortality. Findings on US that are of concern for gangrenous cholecystitis include mucosal ulcerations, sloughed membranes, focal bulge/disrupted wall, and lack of Murphy sign, despite other convincing signs of acute cholecystitis (**Fig. 18**).

Emphysematous Cholecystitis

Emphysematous cholecystitis is a rare condition that is associated with the presence of gas-forming bacteria in the wall of the gallbladder.

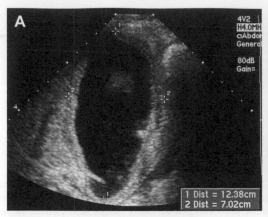
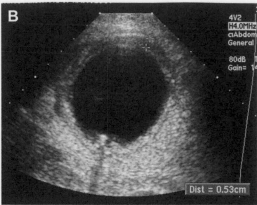

Fig. 15. Acute cholecystitis with gallbladder enlargement. (*A*) Longitudinal view shows an enlarged gallbladder measuring 12.3 × 7.0 cm. (*B*) Transverse view shows a thick wall measuring 5.3 mm and a small stone. (*Data from* Middleton W. General and vascular ultrasound: case review series. Philadelphia: Mosby; 2007. p. 47.)

About 40% of the patients are diabetic. Gallbladder stones are often absent. In these patients, it is thought that cystic artery occlusion caused by inflammation from acute cholecystitis or small vessel atherosclerosis leads to gallbladder wall ischemia, which further leads to overgrowth of gas-producing bacteria. The Clostridia bacteria are most frequently isolated in these instances, with *Clostridium welchii* being the most common.[32] Escherichia coli is isolated with the second most frequency. The mortality rate for acute emphysematous cholecystitis is 15% to 20% (compared to 1.4% for uncomplicated acute cholecystitis), primarily because of a 5-fold increased incidence of gallbladder wall gangrene and perforation.[33] Hence, emphysematous cholecystitis is a surgical emergency requiring prompt

diagnosis and treatment. Definitive treatment is cholecystectomy, but percutaneous cholecystostomy is often used as a temporizing procedure in critically ill patients.

Sonographically, gas in the gallbladder wall appears as a nondependent hyperechoic focus with dirty shadowing or ring-down/comet tail artifact (**Fig. 19**).[34] Associated gas in the lumen may move with changes in the patient's position. Care must be taken to distinguish air in the gallbladder wall from a gallbladder packed with stones or calcification in the gallbladder wall (porcelain gallbladder) because both might appear echogenic with posterior acoustic attenuation. Typically, air produces dirty shadowing, whereas calcification and stones produce clean shadowing. However, there can be an overlap in their sonographic appearance, and in difficult cases, abdominal

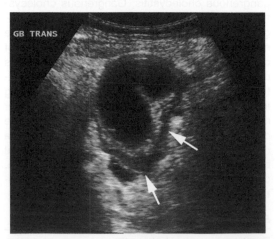

Fig. 16. Acute cholecystitis with pericholecystic fluid. Transverse view shows a slightly folded gallbladder with a localized collection of adjacent fluid (*arrows*).

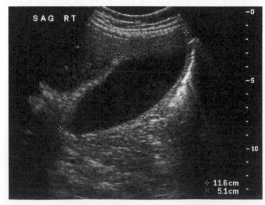

Fig. 17. Acalculous cholecystitis. Longitudinal view shows an enlarged gallbladder measuring 11.6 × 5.1 cm and mild gallbladder wall thickening. No stones were identified.

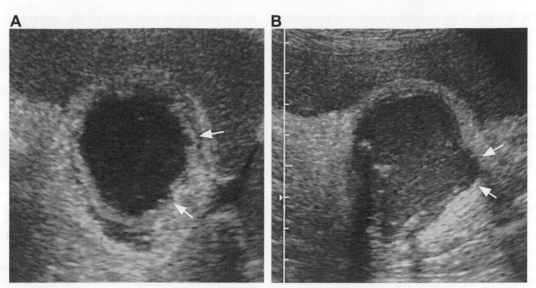

Fig. 18. Gangrenous cholecystitis. (*A*) Magnified transverse view of the gallbladder shows a thick wall with several focal areas of mucosal ulceration (*arrows*). (*B*) Magnified transverse view of the gallbladder in another patient shows a focal bulge in the wall (*arrows*). (*Data from* Middleton W, Kurtz A. Ultrasound: the requisites. 2nd edition. Philadelphia: Mosby; 2004. p. 38.)

radiography and/or CT[35] can allow for definitive distinction between mural gas and calcification. Extensive intramural gas in the gallbladder may mimic the gas-filled bowel and make visualization of the gallbladder impossible. Hence, CT should also be considered in patients with acute RUQ pain in whom the gallbladder is not definitely identified at sonography. Isolated air in the gallbladder lumen can result after recent instrumentation of the biliary tree, such as endoscopic retrograde cholangiopancreatography, placement of biliary stents, or biliary enteric anastomosis, and should not be confused with emphysematous cholecystitis. If iatrogenic causes are excluded, gas in the gallbladder lumen may also indicate a cholecystoenteric fistula.

Gallbladder Perforation

Gallbladder perforation is a serious complication of acute cholecystitis with a mortality rate of

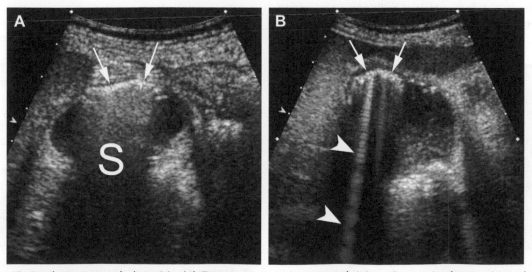

Fig. 19. Emphysematous cholecystitis. (*A*) Transverse view shows very bright reflectors in the nondependent portion of the gallbladder (*arrows*) and an associated dirty shadow (*S*). (*B*) Transverse view shows similar nondependent bright reflectors (*arrows*) and associated ring-down artifact (*arrowheads*).

12% to 16%. This condition occurs in less than 10% of cases of acute cholecystitis. Early detection reduces morbidity and mortality. Predisposing factors for gallbladder perforation include infections, malignancy, steroid therapy, diabetes mellitus, and atherosclerotic heart disease.[36] Niemeier[37] has classified gallbladder perforations into 3 categories: acute, subacute, and chronic. Acute perforation has the worst prognosis because it often results in generalized peritonitis. Subacute perforation is generally contained and often presents with a pericholecystic abscess. Chronic perforation often presents with an internal cholecystic fistula to the duodenum or common bile duct. Most perforations are subacute, accounting for 60% of all cases. Chronic perforations account for 30%, and acute perforations account for 10% of cases. The most common site of perforation is the fundus because it is the most distal part with regard to blood supply. Elderly patients are more susceptible to gallbladder perforation. The incidence of perforation is known to increase 4-fold, with a delay in surgery of more than 2 days from the onset of abdominal symptoms.[38] It may often be difficult to clinically differentiate gallbladder perforation from uncomplicated cholecystitis because the bile leak from a ruptured gallbladder might be contained in the extraperitoneal gallbladder fossa and hence might not produce symptoms of peritonitis immediately.

On sonographic examination, presence of focal bulge, discontinuity, focal intramural fluid collection involving the wall of gallbladder, or a complex pericholecystic fluid collection should raise concern for gallbladder perforation. Visualization of a defect in the gallbladder, also known as hole sign, is a definitive sign of gallbladder perforation (**Fig. 20**).[39] Often, distension of the gallbladder

and edema of its walls may be the earliest signs of impending perforation[40]

SUMMARY

Sonography is the primary imaging modality for the evaluation of RUQ pain. This technique is more effective at diagnosing and evaluating gallstones than any other imaging test. Cholescintigraphy is a valuable test of gallbladder function that is very useful in the evaluation of suspected acute cholecystitis when US is confusing or indeterminate. CT is not a primary modality in the evaluation of RUQ pain but is very useful in further evaluating complicated cholecystitis and gallbladder neoplasms. An understanding of sonographic findings of complications of acute cholecystitis and possible alternative diagnoses aids in prompt diagnosis and appropriate management of patients with RUQ pain.

REFERENCES

1. Hanbidge AE, Buckler PM, O'Malley ME, et al. From the RSNA refresher courses: imaging evaluation for acute pain in the RUQ. Radiographics 2004;24(4):1117–35.
2. Popkharitov AI. Laparoscopic cholecystectomy for acute cholecystitis. Langenbecks Arch Surg 2008; 393(6):935–41.
3. Khan MN, Nordon I, Ghauri AS, et al. Urgent cholecystectomy for acute cholecystitis in a district general hospital—is it feasible? Ann R Coll Surg Engl 2009;91(1):30–4.
4. Gadacz TR. Cholelithiasis and cholecystitis. In: Zuidema GD, editor. Shackelford's surgery of the alimentary tract. 3rd edition. Philadelphia: W.B. Saunders Co; 1991. p. 174–85.
5. Russo MW, Wei JT, Thiny MT, et al. Digestive and liver diseases statistics, 2004. Gastroenterology 2004;126:1448–53.
6. Sandler RS, Everhart JE, Donowitz M, et al. The burden of selected digestive diseases in the United States. Gastroenterology 2002;122:1500–11.
7. Attili AF, Carulli N, Roda E, et al. Epidemiology of gallstone disease in Italy: prevalence data of the Multicenter Italian Study on Cholelithiasis (M.I.COL.). Am J Epidemiol 1995;141:158–65.
8. Everhart JE, Khare M, Hill M, et al. Prevalence and ethnic differences in gallbladder disease in the United States. Gastroenterology 1999;117:632–9.
9. Everhart JE, Yeh F, Lee ET, et al. Prevalence of gallbladder disease in American Indian populations: findings from the Strong Heart Study. Hepatology 2002;35:1507–12.
10. Hopper KD, Landis JR, Meilstrup JW, et al. The prevalence of asymptomatic gallstones in the general population. Invest Radiol 1991;26:939–45.

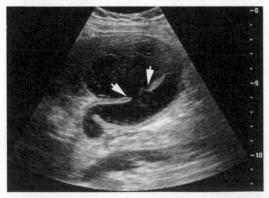

Fig. 20. Gallbladder perforation. Longitudinal view shows a hole in the wall of the gallbladder (*arrows*) with extravasation of luminal contents into the pericholecystic region.

11. Heaton KW, Braddon FE, Mountford RA, et al. Symptomatic and silent gallstones in the community. Gut 1991;32:316–20.

12. Friedman GD, Raviola CA, Fireman B. Prognosis of gallstones with mild or no symptoms: 25 years of follow-up in a health maintenance organization. J Clin Epidemiol 1989;42:127–36.

13. Lee SP, Kuver R. Gallstones. In: Yamada T, editor. Textbook of gastroenterology. 2nd edition. Philadelphia: J.B. Lippincott Co; 1995. p. 2187–212.

14. Trowbridge RL, Rutkowski NK, Shojania KG. Does this patient have acute cholecystitis? JAMA 2003; 289(1):80–6.

15. American College of Radiology appropriateness criteria: RUQ Pain. American College of Radiology. 2010. Available at: http://www.acr.org/Secondary MainMenuCategories/quality_safety/app_criteria/pdf/ ExpertPanelonGastrointestinalImaging/RightUpper QuadrantPainDoc13.aspx. Accessed August 19, 2010.

16. Bennett GL, Balthazar EJ. Ultrasound and CT evaluation of emergent gallbladder pathology. Radiol Clin North Am 2003;41(6):1203–16.

17. Smith EA, Dillman JR, Elsayes KM, et al. Cross-sectional imaging of acute and chronic gallbladder inflammatory disease. AJR Am J Roentgenol 2009; 192(1):188–96.

18. Laing FC, Federle MP, Jeffrey RB, et al. Ultrasonic evaluation of patients with acute RUQ pain. Radiology 1981;140(2):449–55.

19. Ralls PW, Colletti PM, Lapin SA, et al. Real time sonography in suspected acute cholecystitis: prospective evaluation of primary and secondary signs. Radiology 1985;155:767–71.

20. Weissmann HS, Frank MS, Bernstein LH, et al. Rapid and accurate diagnosis of acute cholecystitis with 99m Tc-IDA cholescintigraphy. AJR Am J Roentgenol 1979;132.523–8.

21. Ziessman HA. Acute cholecystitis, biliary obstruction, and biliary leakage. Semin Nucl Med 2003;33: 279–96.

22. Shuman WP, Mack LA, Rudd TG, et al. Evaluation of acute RUQ pain: sonography and 99mTcPIPIDA cholescintigraphy. AJR Am J Roentgenol 1982;139: 61–4.

23. Ralls PW, Colletti PM, Halls JM, et al. Prospective evaluation of 99mTc-IDA cholescintigraphy and gray-scale ultrasound in the diagnosis of acute cholecystitis. Radiology 1982;144:369–71.

24. Worthen NJ, Uszler JM, Funamura JL. Cholecystitis: prospective evaluation of sonography and 99mTc-HIDA cholescintigraphy. AJR 1981;137:973–8.

25. Freitas JE, Mirkes S, Fink-Bennett DM, et al. Suspected acute cholecystitis—comparison of hepatobiliary scintigraphy and ultrasonography. Clin Nucl Med 1982;7:364–7.

26. MacDonald FR, et al. The WES triad—a specific sonographic sign of stones in the contracted gallbladder. Gastrointest Radiol 1981;6:39–41.

27. Raghavendra BN, Subramanyam BR, Balthazar EJ, et al. Sonography of adenomyomatosis of the gallbladder: radiologic-pathologic correlation. Radiology 1983;146:747–52.

28. Soyer P, Brouland JP, Boudiaf M, et al. Color velocity imaging and power Doppler sonography of the gallbladder wall: a new look at sonographic diagnosis of acute cholecystitis. AJR Am J Roentgenol 1998;171: 183–8.

29. Barie PS, Eachempati SR. Acute acalculous cholecystitis. Gastroenterol Clin North Am 2010;39(2): 343–57.

30. Jeffrey RB, Laing FC, Wong W, et al. Gangrenous cholecystitis: diagnosis by ultrasound. Radiology 1983;148:219–21.

31. Simeone JF, Brink JA, Mueller PR, et al. The sonographic diagnosis of acute gangrenous cholecystitis: importance of the Murphy sign. AJR Am J Roentgenol 1989;152(2):289–90.

32. Garcia-Sancho Tellez L, Rodriquez,-Montes JA, Fernandez de Lis S, et al. Acute emphysematous cholecystitis. Report of twenty cases. Hepatogastroenterology 1999;46:2144–214.

33. Mentzer RM Jr, Golden GT, Chandler JG, et al. A comparative appraisal of emphysematous cholecystitis. Am J Surg 1975;129:10–5.

34. Bloom RA, Libson E, Lebensart PD, et al. The ultrasound spectrum of emphysematous cholecystitis. J Clin Ultrasound 1989;17:251–6.

35. Grayson DE, Abbott RM, Levy AD, et al. Emphysematous infections of the abdomen and pelvis: a pictorial review. Radiographics 2002;22:543–61.

36. Derici H, Kara C, Bozdag AD, et al. Diagnosis and treatment of gallbladder perforation. World J Gastroenterol 2006;12:7832–6.

37. Niemeier OW. Acute free perforation of the gallbladder. Ann Surg 1934;99:922–4.

38. Harland C, Mayberry JF, Toghill PJ. Type 1 free perforation of the gallbladder. J R Soc Med 1985;78:725–8.

39. Sood BP, Kalra N, Gupta S, et al. Role of sonography in the diagnosis of gallbladder perforation. J Clin Ultrasound 2002;30:270–4.

40. Soiva M, Pamilo M, Päivänsalo M, et al. Ultrasonography in acute gallbladder perforation. Acta Radiol 1988;29:41–4.

Acute Pelvic Pain in Women: Ultrasonography Still Reigns

Sheila Sheth, MD

KEYWORDS

- Acute pelvic pain • Pelvic inflammatory disease
- Ultrasonography • Torsion

Acute pelvic pain is one of the most common symptoms prompting women to seek emergent care. And yet, because clinical signs of the various underlying causes overlap, accurate diagnosis is often elusive without appropriate history, laboratory tests, and imaging. The most common conditions presenting acutely include ectopic pregnancy; spontaneous abortion in pregnant women; and ovarian cysts, ovarian torsion, and pelvic inflammatory disease (PID) in nongravid patients. Nongynecologic disorders such as acute appendicitis and ureteral colic can also present with pain referred to the lower abdomen.

Imaging allows rapid and often precise diagnosis, leading to an optimal management, especially allowing efficient triaging of patients between medical or symptomatic treatment, gynecologic consultation or referral to surgery, and interventional radiology. Despite the presence of multidetector row computed tomography (CT) in an increasing number of emergency departments, ultrasonography (US) remains the best imaging modality for these patients. High-resolution endovaginal probes allow exquisite visualization and characterization of the pelvic organs and can be used to great advantage in confirming that an abnormality is indeed the source of the woman's symptoms if gentle pressure from the probe precipitates focal tenderness. Lack of ionizing radiation is another significant advantage over CT, particularly because most patients are women of reproductive age. US has a limited field of view, however, and the sonographer or sonologist should make certain that the area of pain is thoroughly examined, regardless of the study requested.

This article discusses gynecologic diseases presenting with acute or subacute pelvic pain and presents some other causes of pelvic pain that may mimic gynecologic disorders. Ectopic pregnancy is discussed elsewhere and will not be addressed.

COMPLICATIONS OF FUNCTIONAL OVARIAN CYSTS

Sudden hemorrhage within a functional ovarian cyst or leakage of cyst fluid within the cul-de-sac can present acutely with severe lower abdominal pain. Follicular cysts result from the failure of a dominant follicle to expel its oocyte. They are easily diagnosed as an anechoic intraovarian lesion with thin walls and increased through transmission. Corpus lutei and corpus luteal cysts are particularly prone to hemorrhage and rupture because of the normal neovascularity in their wall. Functional ovarian cysts resolve spontaneously within 1 or 2 menstrual cycles.

US Findings

Hemorrhagic ovarian cysts display characteristic sonographic appearances, allowing for confident diagnosis and conservative management.

The sonographic findings vary with the age of the hemorrhage (**Figs. 1** and **2**).[1] Whereas fresh blood is anechoic, subacute intracystic hemorrhage is hyperechoic or isoechoic to the ovarian

Johns Hopkins Medical Institutions, Baltimore, MD, USA
E-mail address: ssheth@jhmi.edu

Ultrasound Clin 6 (2011) 163–176
doi:10.1016/j.cult.2011.03.006

ultrasound.theclinics.com

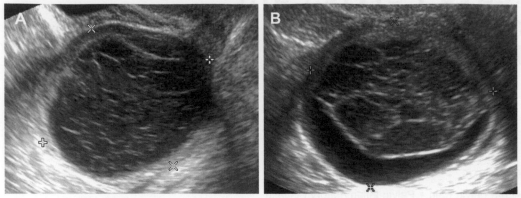

Fig. 1. Classic US appearances of hemorrhagic ovarian cysts in 2 different patients. (*A*) Sagittal EVUS of the left ovary shows a fine reticular or lace-like pattern within a cystic lesion. (*B*) Sagittal EVUS of the right ovary shows a retracting clot with straight or concave borders. EVUS, endovaginal ultrasonography.

stroma and may be difficult to distinguish from an ovarian mass without a follow-up sonography. As the clot forms, fibrin stranding within the cyst appears as a fine reticular fishnet or lace-like pattern. The reticular pattern differs from true septations in an ovarian neoplasm, which are more echogenic and less numerous. An intracystic mass with triangular or concave borders and without blood flow is seen as the clot retracts and should not be mistaken for a nodule within an ovarian neoplasm. The reticular pattern or retracting clot is seen in 90% of hemorrhagic cysts. Thus, the presence of either sign in an ovarian lesion greatly increases the likelihood that it is a hemorrhagic cyst, allowing for confident diagnosis and conservative management.[2] Follow-up with imaging is not necessary if the findings are classic, provided the size of the lesion is 5 cm or less.[3] However, if the appearance of the lesion is atypical, short-term follow-up US in 6 weeks should be recommended because hemorrhagic cysts should decrease in size or resolve. Pelvic MR imaging should only be obtained for the rare hemorrhagic cyst that mimics an ovarian neoplasm (**Fig. 3**).

Ruptured Ovarian Cyst

Rupture of an ovarian cyst can be inferred if there is complex free fluid in the pelvis and there is a collapsed cyst with crenated borders within the ovary (**Fig. 4**). Much less commonly, the hemorrhage resulting from the ruptured cyst can be massive, resulting in symptoms and signs of

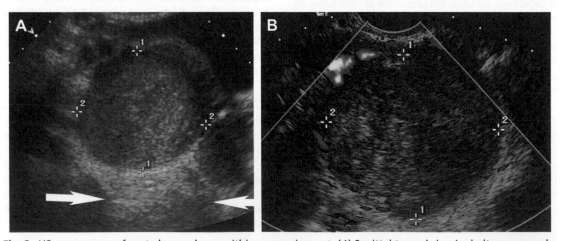

Fig. 2. US appearance of acute hemorrhage within an ovarian cyst. (*A*) Sagittal transabdominal ultrasonography shows an echogenic mass within the right ovary. There is some mass through transmission (*arrows*), suggesting that the mass is cystic. (*B*) Sagittal endovaginal ultrasonography of the right ovary shows the echogenic lesion with no intrinsic flow on power Doppler. The lesion resolved on follow-up US 5 weeks later, confirming the diagnosis.

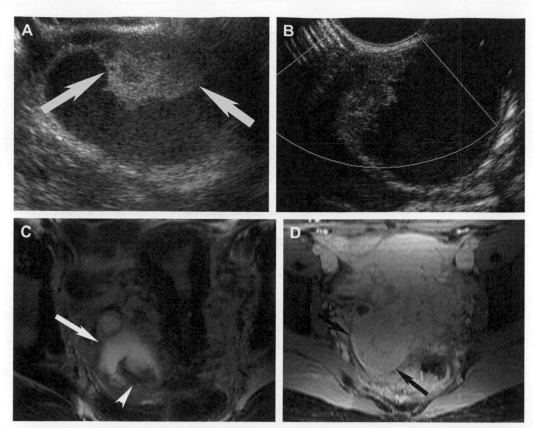

Fig. 3. Hemorrhagic cyst mimicking ovarian neoplasm. MR imaging was obtained because of the appearance of the lesion in a woman with a family history of ovarian cancer. (*A*) Sagittal EVUS of the right ovary shows a complex cystic mass with an echogenic component suspicious for mural nodule (*arrows*). (*B*) Coronal EVUS of the right ovary with color Doppler shows absence of flow within the echogenic component. (*C*) Axial T2-weighted MR imaging of the pelvis shows a cystic lesion within the right ovary (*arrow*) with T2 dark material in its dependent portion (*arrowhead*). (*D*) Axial postcontrast MR imaging shows no enhancement within the lesion. The MR imaging appearance is consistent with a hemorrhagic cyst, and the lesion resolved on follow-up. EVUS, endovaginal ultrasonography.

hypovolemia clinically and hemoperitoneum on imaging. The ovary may be surrounded by organized clots and difficult to identify, and the collapsed cyst may be undetected unless carefully sought on vaginal US (**Fig. 5**).[4] Although rupture does occur spontaneously, patients on anticoagulation therapy are at a higher risk (**Fig. 6**). The main challenge is to differentiate this condition from a ruptured ectopic pregnancy so that correlation with urine or serum human chorionic gonadotropin is mandatory. However, concurrent intrauterine pregnancy and ruptured corpus luteum have been reported.

Ovarian and Adnexal Endometrioma

Endometriosis, the implantation of endometrial tissue outside the uterus, usually manifests itself as chronic pelvic pain, dysmenorrhea, or infertility. However, occasionally ovarian endometriomas,

the so-called chocolate cyst, can present acutely or rupture and cause hemoperitoneum. Although endometrial implants cannot be detected on US, endometriomas have a characteristic appearance of unilocular or multilocular cystic mass filled with low-level echoes (**Fig. 7**).[5] Small bright echogenic foci in the wall of the cysts are highly suggestive of the diagnosis and are thought to be caused by cell breakdown products.[6]

ADNEXAL TORSION

Adnexal torsion, or twisting of the fallopian tube and/or the ovary around the vascular pedicle of the ovary, leads to permanent ischemic damage to the affected ovary unless the condition is diagnosed early and relieved by emergent surgical detorsion before hemorrhagic infarction of the ovary develops.

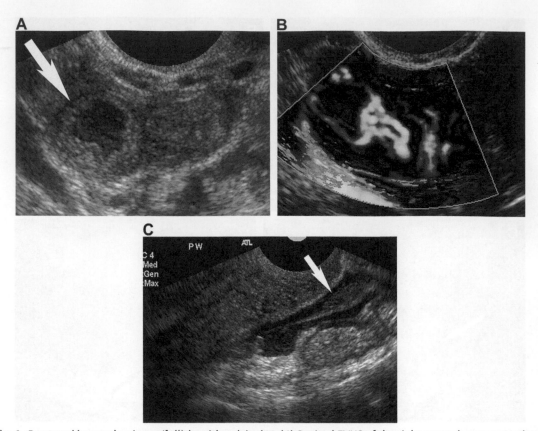

Fig. 4. Ruptured hemorrhagic cyst/follicle with pelvic clot. (*A*) Sagittal EVUS of the right ovary shows a crenulated small complex cystic lesion compatible with a collapsing corpus luteum (*arrow*). (*B*) On power Doppler US, neovascularity around the corpus luteum is noted. (*C*) Sagittal EVUS of the cul-de-sac shows blood and organized clots (*arrow*). EVUS, endovaginal ultrasonography.

In young girls, the torsion is often spontaneous. Adnexal torsion most commonly affects women of reproductive age with an underlying ovarian mass, a large cyst, or a cystic teratoma, acting as a fulcrum in up to half of the patients.[7] In postmenopausal women, adnexal torsion is uncommon but associated with an ovarian mass in more than 80% of patients.[7]

Patients usually present with severe pelvic pain, nausea, and a surgical abdomen. Gynecologic examination may be limited because of extreme patient discomfort, and imaging plays a critical role in the diagnosis.

US Findings

The sonographic appearance of adnexal torsion on gray scale reflects the underlying pathologic changes.

Enlargement of the ovary is the most common finding because of edema and congestion caused by obstruction of venous return. If the adnexal pedicle is tightly twisted or if the condition progresses, arterial occlusion and ischemia follow. In most patients the authors have observed, the ovarian tissue has heterogeneous echotexture because of ischemia and hemorrhage and the ovary is usually necrotic and nonviable at surgery. An ovarian mass, commonly a large cyst or cystic teratoma, can be present (**Fig. 8**). The classic enlarged ovary with peripheral follicles is seen in a few cases (**Fig. 9**).

The adnexal mass is often in an unusual location, either in the cul-de-sac or above the uterus.

Direct visualization of the twisted adnexal pedicle should be attempted. Lee and colleagues[8] were able to detect the twisted pedicle in most of their patients with surgically proven torsion, for a diagnostic accuracy of 87%. On the gray scale, the twisted adnexal pedicle appears as a round mass with concentric hypoechoic and echogenic stripes located between the uterus and the enlarged adnexa.[8] The whirlpool sign refers to direct observation of the coiled vessels within the twisted adnexal pedicle on color Doppler and has been associated with a high degree of

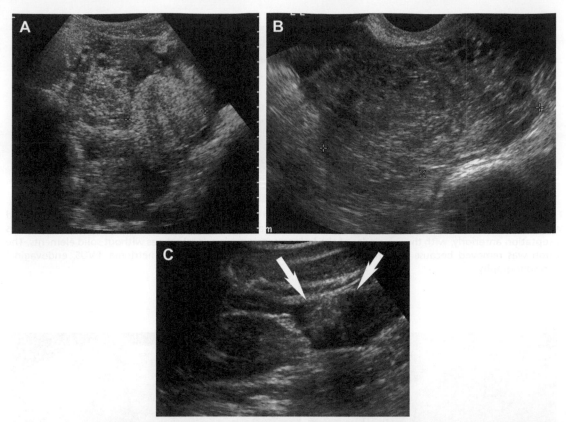

Fig. 5. Ruptured hemorrhagic cyst with hemoperitoneum and clots in the right adnexa. (*A*) Transverse TAUS of the pelvis shows large amount of complex amorphous material compatible with clot surrounding the uterus. (*B*) Sagittal endovaginal ultrasonography of the right adnexa shows a complex amorphous mass with no recognizable ovarian tissue. (*C*) Sagittal TAUS of the right flank shows complex fluid compatible with hemoperitoneum. The patient had a negative human chorionic gonadotropin, was hemodynamically stable, and treated conservatively. Follow-up US showed resolution of the findings. TAUS, transabdominal ultrasonography.

specificity: in a retrospective study, the whirlpool sign was seen in 20 of 22 women with surgically proven adnexal torsion (**Fig. 10**).[9] However, this study does not address the sensitivity of the whirlpool sign, and its absence cannot exclude the diagnosis if other sonographic findings strongly suggest torsion. In addition, this sign needs to be carefully sought by moving the

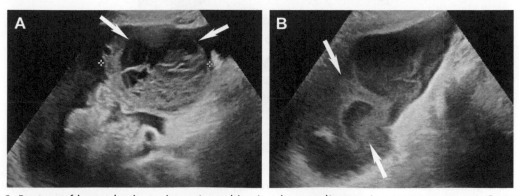

Fig. 6. Rupture of hemorrhagic ovarian cyst, resulting in a hemoperitoneum in a young woman on Coumadin (anticoagulation therapy). (*A*) Transverse TAUS of the right lower quadrant shows a classic hemorrhagic right ovarian cyst (*arrows*). Note the complex fluid in the right lower quadrant. (*B*) Transverse TAUS of the right lower quadrant more laterally shows clots within the right lower quadrant (*arrows*). TAUS, transabdominal ultrasonography.

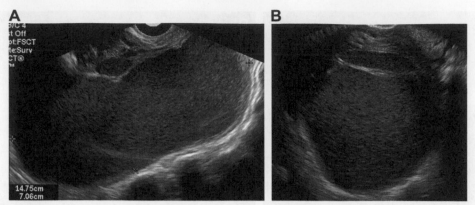

Fig. 7. Large ovarian endometrioma. (A) Sagittal EVUS of the right adnexa shows a large cystic adnexal mass filled with diffuse low-level echoes, a sonographic pattern called a ground glass appearance. (B) Coronal EVUS shows a septation anteriorly, with the remainder of the lesion containing low-level echoes without solid elements. The lesion was removed because of patient discomfort and proved to be an endometrioma. EVUS, endovaginal ultrasonography.

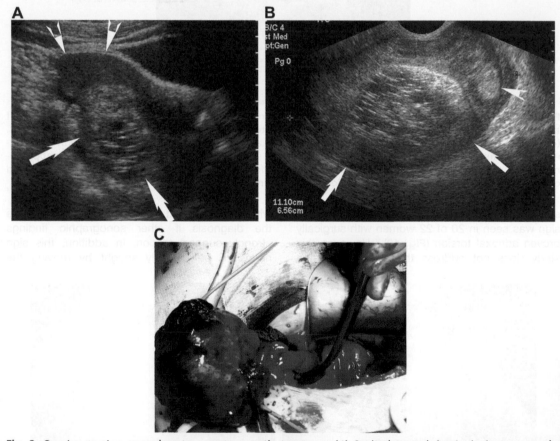

Fig. 8. Ovarian torsion secondary to a mature cystic teratoma. (A) Sagittal transabdominal ultrasonography shows a large heterogeneous mass in the cul-de-sac (arrows), posterior to the uterus (arrowhead). (B) Sagittal endovaginal ultrasonography shows a very large ovary in an abnormal position in the cul-de-sac. There is a mixed cystic and solid mass containing multiple echogenic linear interfaces, characteristic of a dermoid mesh (arrows). The rest of the ovarian parenchyma is heterogeneous with areas of hemorrhage (arrowhead). The patient was extremely tender during the examination. No Doppler flow could be elicited from the mass. (C) Intraoperative twisted adnexal pedicle and necrotic enlarged ovary.

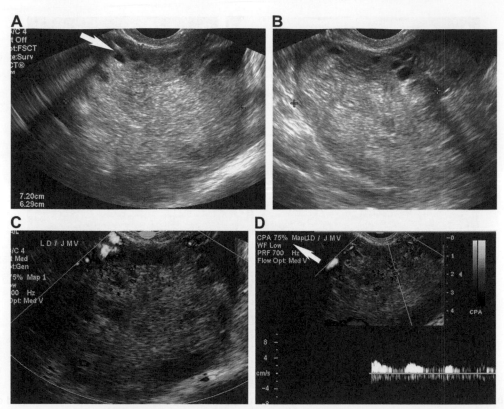

Fig. 9. Ovarian torsion. (*A*) Sagittal EVUS of the right ovary shows a markedly enlarged ovary with heterogeneous echogenic stroma and peripheral follicles. (*B*) Transverse EVUS of the right ovary confirms the findings. (*C*) Sagittal EVUS of the right ovary with power Doppler shows minimal flow at the periphery of the ovary. (*D*) Doppler spectrum shows minimal arterial flow within the ovary. Note that the Doppler parameters have been optimized for low-flow settings (*arrow*). EVUS, endovaginal ultrasonography.

transducer along the axis of the adnexal pedicle (see **Fig. 10**).

Color, power, and spectral Doppler evaluations of the ovary yield variable results, and some authors have suggested that intraovarian blood flow analysis may be helpful to predict viability or irreversible ischemic changes in the ovary. The latter condition is suspected when there is absence of any arterial or venous flow within the ovary, and surgery usually confirms the presence of necrosis. Absence of venous flow within the ovary is also highly predictive of torsion and can be seen with milder degree of twisting.[10] However, the gray-scale findings are most important because normal blood flow has been detected in surgically proven cases, perhaps related to intermittent torsion or the presence of a dual ovarian blood supply.

PELVIC INFLAMMATORY DISEASE

PID is the most common cause of acute pelvic pain in women of reproductive age. It refers to

a sexually transmitted infection of the upper genital tract. The infection, most commonly caused by *Chlamydia trachomatis* or *Neisseria gonorrhoeae*, spreads along the uterine cervix and the endometrium to the fallopian tube, the surface of the ovaries, and the peritoneal cavity. Women with a history of sexually transmitted diseases and multiple sexual partners and sexually active adolescent girls are particularly at risk for PID. Recent placement of an intrauterine contraceptive device seems to be a significant precipitating factor. Less common causes of pelvic infection include direct spread from the gastrointestinal tract, acute appendicitis, diverticulitis, or Crohn abscesses. Hematogenous spread is much less common but can be seen in patients with tuberculosis.

PID affects approximately 10% to 15% of women in the United States and represents a significant threat to their well-being because the long-term sequelae of PID include infertility, chronic pain, and ectopic pregnancy.[11]

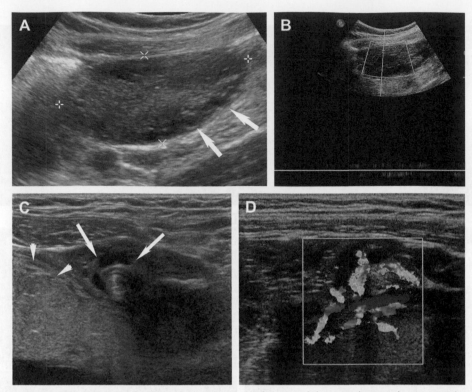

Fig. 10. Ovarian torsion in a woman 22 weeks' pregnant with twins. (*A*) Sagittal TAUS shows an enlarged ovary (the ovary measured 6.0 × 2.4 × 4 cm) with peripheral follicles (*arrows*). The patient was focally tender over the ovary. (*B*) Power Doppler image of the ovary shows only a minimal amount of flow within the ovary. Because the Doppler spectral signal is displayed symmetrically on both sides of the baseline, the signal may be artifactual rather than representing true flow. (*C*) Transverse TAUS shows a small round lesion with a target appearance (*arrows*) between the abnormal ovary and the uterus (*arrowhead*), representing the twisted adnexal pedicle. (*D*) Color Doppler image over this area shows the whirlpool sign of twisted vessels. Ovarian torsion was confirmed at surgery. TAUS, transabdominal ultrasonography.

The symptoms and signs of PID include pelvic pain, fever, foul smelling vaginal discharge, and cervical motion tenderness. However, these symptoms are nonspecific, and US is usually requested to confirm the diagnosis and help in patient management by detecting severe PID requiring percutaneous or surgical drainage.

US Findings

In patients with mild or early PID, the US findings may be absent or subtle, with mild enlargement of the uterus and ovaries and ill-defined tissue planes in the pelvis. These findings may be only evident in retrospect and better appreciated on transabdominal US because of its wider field of view.[12] Visualization of mildly enlarged ovaries with peripheral small follicles and prominent stroma, mimicking polycystic ovaries, has been suggested as an early sign of PID (**Fig. 11**).[13] The presence of a thickened endometrial complex or endometrial fluid suggests endometritis. Complex

free pelvic fluid is seen if there is free pus in the pelvis.

The most important sonographic abnormalities relate to the fallopian tubes and usually affect both sides. Salpingitis manifests a thickening of 5 mm or more of the normally imperceptible wall of the tube. When seen in cross section, the thickened endosalpingeal folds appear as the classic cog wheel. This sign is thought to be specific for acute tubal inflammation.[11] As the infection progresses, distal occlusion leads to the formation of pyosalpinx, easily recognized on endovaginal scanning (EVS) as a tubular adnexal mass with thick walls, incomplete septations containing complex fluid, or a fluid debris level (**Fig. 12**). In severe cases, the acutely inflamed fallopian tube becomes adherent to the ovary and cannot be separated by gentle pressure from the EVS probe. In classic PID, the process is usually bilateral, the so-called tubo-ovarian complex. The most advanced form of PID is the tubo-ovarian abscess; a large, complex, and acutely tender adnexal

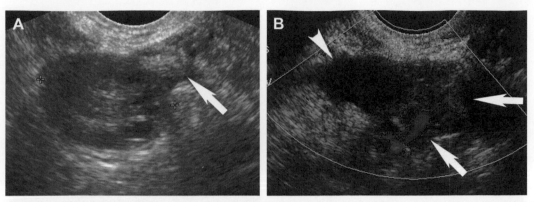

Fig. 11. Subtle US findings in mild PID. (*A*) Coronal EVUS of the right adnexa shows a minimally thickened right fallopian tube, medial to the right ovary (*arrow*). Note the prominent ovarian stroma. (*B*) Sagittal color Doppler EVUS shows some hyperemia within the wall of the thickened right fallopian tube (*arrows*). There is some free fluid seen (*arrowhead*). EVUS, endovaginal ultrasonography.

mass engulfs the tube and the ovary with destruction of the normal architecture (**Fig. 13**).

Color and power Doppler show an increase in vascularity around the adnexal mass, reflecting hyperemia of acute inflammation. These Doppler findings are most helpful in mild or equivocal cases of salpingitis before the formation of pyosalpinx (see **Fig. 11**).[14]

The adnexal findings are often outlined by increased echogenicity of the adjacent mesenteric fat. Hyperechoic fat is associated with acute infection or inflammation anywhere in the abdomen, which is the sonographic equivalent of the mesenteric standing seen on CT, and it is found to be a useful secondary sign.

NONGYNECOLOGIC CAUSES OF ACUTE PELVIC PAIN

Besides the uterus, fallopian tubes, and ovaries, the female pelvis is home to the loops of small bowel, portions of the colon, the bladder, and the distal ureters. Many of the pathologic processes affecting these structures also present with pain, mimic a gynecologic emergency, and, in some cases, lie within the reach of the endovaginal probe. In these cases, although CT remains the primary imaging modality and will be requested to confirm or clarify the US findings, once again the real-time and interactive capabilities of US are valuable, particularly in young thin patients with minimal amount of pelvic mesenteric fat.

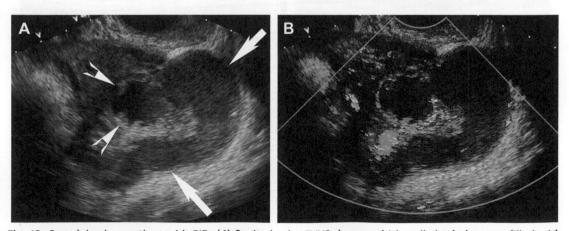

Fig. 12. Pyosalpinx in a patient with PID. (*A*) Sagittal color EVUS shows a thick-walled tubular mass filled with internal echoes consistent with a pyosalpinx (*arrows*). Note the cogwheel appearance of thickened folds seen in cross section (*arrowhead*) and the echogenic fat around the pyosalpinx. (*B*) Sagittal color Doppler EVUS shows hyperemia within the wall of the pyosalpinx. EVUS, endovaginal ultrasonography.

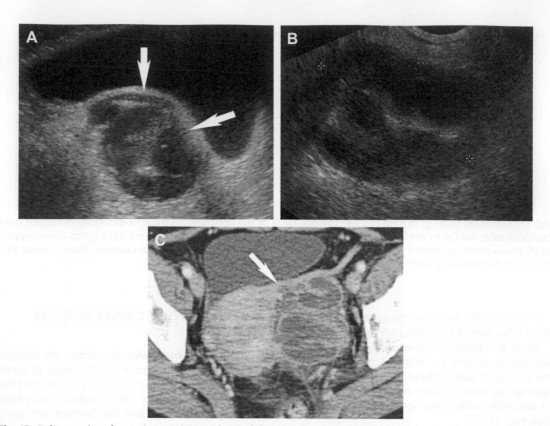

Fig. 13. Tubo-ovarian abscess in a patient with PID. (*A*) Sagittal transabdominal ultrasonography shows a complex left adnexal mass with thick walls and internal echoes (*arrow*). (*B*) Coronal endovaginal ultrasonography of the left adnexa confirms the findings. The left ovary could not be identified separately. (*C*) Axial CT of the pelvis with intravenous contrast shows a left adnexal mass with enhancing septations (*arrow*).

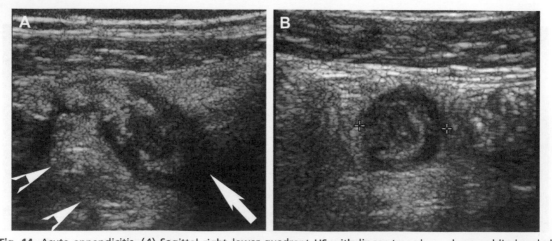

Fig. 14. Acute appendicitis. (*A*) Sagittal right–lower quadrant US with linear transducer shows a blind-ended noncompressible loop of bowel, compatible with acute appendicitis (*arrow*). Note the surrounding echogenic fat and indication of inflammation The patient was extremely tender on palpation of the appendix by the US transducer. (*B*) Transverse right–lower quadrant US shows the symmetrically thickened appendiceal wall.

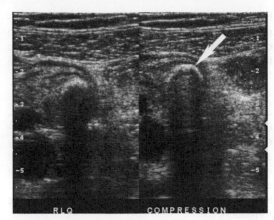

Fig. 15. Acute appendicitis with appendicolith. Sagittal right–lower quadrant US with linear transducer shows a blind-ended noncompressible loop of bowel, compatible with acute appendicitis (*arrow*). There is an echogenic focus with distal acoustic shadowing near the tip of the appendix (*arrow*).

Acute Appendicitis

Classic clinical findings associated with acute appendicitis include abdominal pain, migrating from the periumbilical area to the right lower quadrant over the course of several hours; nausea; and low-grade fever. Although the clinical criteria to diagnose acute appendicitis are well established, there is a significant overlap with other conditions, particularly with PID and ovarian torsion. To minimize the number of unnecessary appendectomies, confirmation of the diagnosis with imaging, either CT or US, has gained wide acceptance,[15] particularly in women of reproductive age who have been shown to benefit the most from preoperative imaging.[16]

US findings

The technique of graded compression US to diagnose acute appendicitis, first described by Puylaert,[17] has now been validated by multiple other studies. Using a linear or curvilinear transducer, the sonographer or sonologist examines the right lower quadrant by applying gradually increasing pressure over the cecum. The normal bowel and appendix should compress without eliciting significant pain. By contrast, the diagnosis of acute appendicitis rests on the demonstration of a noncompressible blind-ending loop measuring more than 6 mm (**Fig. 14**).[18] The presence of an appendicolith (**Fig. 15**), focal tenderness, and guarding under the transducer are additional important signs. The fat surrounding the appendix becomes echogenic, which may facilitate detection of the abnormal appendix, and color or power Doppler often demonstrates hyperemia in the appendiceal wall (**Fig. 16**). It is important to examine the entire appendix to avoid missing tip appendicitis. Pelvic US, which is often requested in conjunction with right lower quadrant because of the overlap of clinical findings with gynecologic conditions, may show complex pelvic fluid. Occasionally, if the appendix is located in the pelvis, US findings of appendicitis are exquisitely displayed on endovaginal ultrasonography. The classic gut signature of alternating echogenic and hypoechoic layers of the thickened appendix allows its differentiation from an abnormal fallopian tube (see **Fig. 16**).

There are significant limitations to graded compression US for the diagnosis of appendicitis, with a mean sensitivity of 78% and specificity of 83% compared with contrast-enhanced CT with a sensitivity of 91% and specificity of 90%, as reported in a recent meta-analysis.[19] These

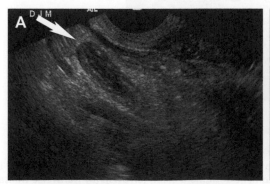
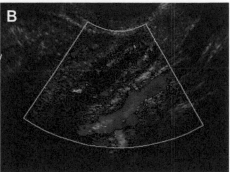

Fig. 16. Acute appendicitis seen on EVUS. (*A*) Sagittal EVUS of the right adnexa shows a blind-ending loop with typical gut signature (*arrow*). The patient was exquisitely tender over that area. (*B*) Sagittal EVUS of the right adnexa with color Doppler shows hyperemia within the wall of the thickened appendix. EVUS, endovaginal ultrasonography.

limitations include large body habitus, operator experience, and atypical location of the appendix in retrocecal region or deep in the pelvis.

US is also more limited than CT in the diagnosis of perforated appendix, although this complication should be suspected if there is a break in the echogenic submucosal ring of the appendix.[20]

Diverticulitis

Acute diverticulitis results from an inflammation of colonic diverticula obstructed by inspissated fecal material. It commonly results in focal microperforation or macroperforation. Complications include local abscess formation or fistulous tract.

US findings

Acute diverticulitis appears as a focal thickening of a segment of colon caused by muscular

hypertrophy and pericolonic inflammation evidenced by echogenic fat. The ruptured diverticula can sometimes be visualized as bright echogenic foci with ring-down artifacts seen beyond the confines of the thickened bowel wall (**Fig. 17**).[21]

Crohn Disease

Crohn disease is a chronic granulomatous inflammatory disease of unknown cause most frequently affecting the terminal ileum and the cecum. It is characterized by recurrent episodes of acute inflammation alternating with period of remissions, leading to bowel strictures, fistula, and abscess formation.

US findings

Barium studies and CT are the preferred imaging modalities in patients with Crohn disease. However, some patients present with an acute

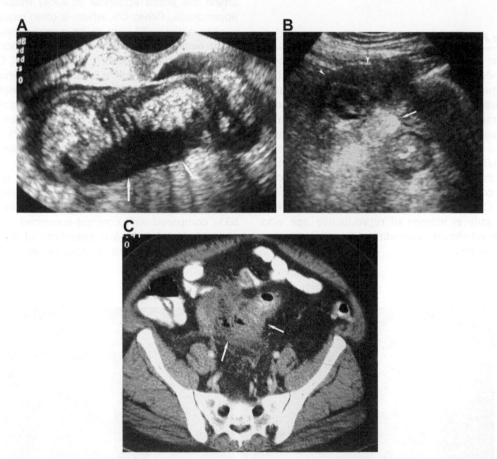

Fig. 17. Acute diverticulitis with focal perforation in a patient with suspected PID. (*A*) Sagittal endovaginal ultrasonography of the left pelvis shows a thick-walled segment of sigmoid colon (*arrows*). (*B*) Transverse transabdominal ultrasonography over the pelvis shows an ill-defined fluid collection (*arrowheads*). There are echogenic foci with dirty shadowing that appears extraluminal. Diverticulitis with focal perforation was suspected, and the patient had a CT scan with contrast. (*C*) Axial CT with contrast shows thickening of the sigmoid colon with extraluminal air and mesenteric stranding, confirming the diagnosis.

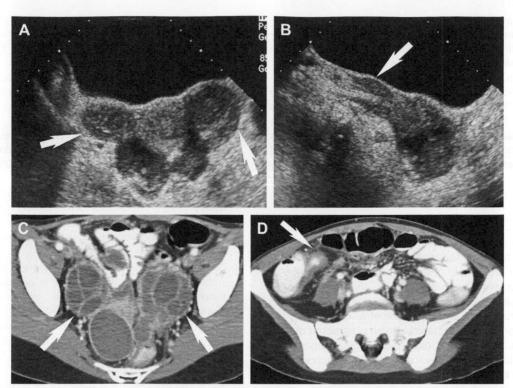

Fig. 18. Acute presentation of Crohn disease with pelvic abscesses and fistula. (*A*) Transverse TAUS of the pelvis shows complex fluid collections in both adnexae (*arrows*). (*B*) Sagittal TAUS shows linear hypoechoic tracts suggesting fistulae (*arrows*). (*C*) Axial CT with contrast shows bilateral pelvic fluid collections with enhancing walls (*arrows*). (*D*) Axial CT with contrast shows thickening of the distal ileum (*arrow*) compatible with Crohn ileitis. TAUS, transabdominal ultrasonography.

episode of lower abdominal pain mimicking a gynecologic disorder.

US can demonstrate thick bowel wall, enlarged reactive lymph nodes, abscesses, and fistula formation and can be useful to differentiate drainable fluid collections from phlegmons (**Fig. 18**).[22]

SPECIAL CLINICAL SCENARIOS
Acute Pelvic Pain in Pregnancy

Acute pelvic pain in pregnant women poses specific diagnostic and management challenges. As the gravid uterus displaces pelvic organs, imaging with US may be more difficult and pelvic

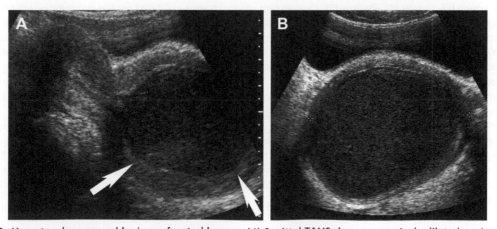

Fig. 19. Hematocolpos caused by imperforated hymen. (*A*) Sagittal TAUS shows a massively dilated vagina filled with low-level echoes (*arrows*). (*B*) Transverse TAUS confirms the findings. TAUS, transabdominal ultrasonography.

MR imaging is a valuable adjunct as a problem-solving tool. If an acute surgical abdomen is suspected, CT is justified despite the risk of radiation to the fetus to expedite the care of the patient.[23]

Acute appendicitis is the most common nonobstetric surgical emergency in pregnancy affecting 1 of 1500 pregnancies, and symptoms and signs may be atypical. Ovarian torsion can complicate an otherwise normal pregnancy. Uterine fibroids are an uncommon cause of pain in the nongravid patient, but they can occasionally present acutely in pregnancy if they outgrow their blood supply and undergo rapid degeneration.

Pelvic Pain in Teenagers

After the onset of menarche, causes of acute pelvic pain in teenage girls are similar to those in older women. In girls with primary amenorrhea or oligomenorrhea, one should also consider the possibility of an imperforate hymen with hematometrocolpos and hematometra or a mullerian abnormality associated with an obstructed uterine horn. On US, the distended vagina appears as a midline mass filled with low-level echoes and with thick smooth walls (**Fig. 19**).

REFERENCES

1. Jain KA. Sonographic spectrum of hemorrhagic ovarian cysts. J Ultrasound Med 2002;21:879–86.
2. Patel MD, Feldstein VA, Filly RA. The likelihood ratio of sonographic findings for the diagnosis of hemorrhagic ovarian cysts. J Ultrasound Med 2005;24: 607–14 [quiz: 15].
3. Levine D, Brown DL, Andreotti RF, et al. Management of asymptomatic ovarian and other adnexal cysts imaged at US: Society of Radiologists in Ultrasound Consensus Conference Statement. Radiology 2010;256:943–54.
4. Hertzberg BS, Kliewer MA, Paulson EK. Ovarian cyst rupture causing hemoperitoneum: imaging features and the potential for misdiagnosis. Abdom Imaging 1999;24:304–8.
5. Asch E, Levine D. Variations in appearance of endometriomas. J Ultrasound Med 2007;26:993–1002.
6. Patel MD, Feldstein VA, Chen DC, et al. Endometriomas: diagnostic performance of US. Radiology 1999;210:739–45.
7. Chiou SY, Lev-Toaff AS, Masuda E, et al. Adnexal torsion: new clinical and imaging observations by sonography, computed tomography, and magnetic resonance imaging. J Ultrasound Med 2007;26: 1289–301.
8. Lee EJ, Kwon HC, Joo HJ, et al. Diagnosis of ovarian torsion with color Doppler sonography: depiction of twisted vascular pedicle. J Ultrasound Med 1998; 17:83–9.
9. Valsky DV, Esh-Broder E, Cohen SM, et al. Added value of the gray-scale whirlpool sign in the diagnosis of adnexal torsion. Ultrasound Obstet Gynecol 2010;36:630–4.
10. Auslender R, Shen O, Kaufman Y, et al. Doppler and gray-scale sonographic classification of adnexal torsion. Ultrasound Obstet Gynecol 2009;34:208–11.
11. Timor-Tritsch IE, Lerner JP, Monteagudo A, et al. Transvaginal sonographic markers of tubal inflammatory disease. Ultrasound Obstet Gynecol 1998; 12:56–66.
12. Horrow MM. Ultrasound of pelvic inflammatory disease. Ultrasound Q 2004;20:171–9.
13. Cacciatore B, Leminen A, Ingman-Friberg S, et al. Transvaginal sonographic findings in ambulatory patients with suspected pelvic inflammatory disease. Obstet Gynecol 1992;80:912–6.
14. Molander P, Sjoberg J, Paavonen J, et al. Transvaginal power Doppler findings in laparoscopically proven acute pelvic inflammatory disease. Ultrasound Obstet Gynecol 2001;17:233–8.
15. Toorenvliet BR, Wiersma F, Bakker RF, et al. Routine ultrasound and limited computed tomography for the diagnosis of acute appendicitis. World J Surg 2010;34:2278–85.
16. Bendeck SE, Nino-Murcia M, Berry GJ, et al. Imaging for suspected appendicitis: negative appendectomy and perforation rates. Radiology 2002;225:131–6.
17. Puylaert JB. Ultrasound of acute GI tract conditions. Eur Radiol 2001;11:1867–77.
18. Jeffrey RB Jr, Laing FC, Townsend RR. Acute appendicitis: sonographic criteria based on 250 cases. Radiology 1988;167:327–9.
19. van Randen A, Bipat S, Zwinderman AH, et al. Acute appendicitis: meta-analysis of diagnostic performance of CT and graded compression US related to prevalence of disease. Radiology 2008;249:97–106.
20. Jeffrey RB, Jain KA, Nghiem HV. Sonographic diagnosis of acute appendicitis: interpretive pitfalls. AJR Am J Roentgenol 1994;162:55–9.
21. Wilson SR, Toi A. The value of sonography in the diagnosis of acute diverticulitis of the colon. AJR Am J Roentgenol 1990;154:1199–202.
22. Sturm EJ, Cobben LP, Meijssen MA, et al. Detection of ileocecal Crohn's disease using ultrasound as the primary imaging modality. Eur Radiol 2004;14:778–82.
23. Kilpatrick CC, Monga M. Approach to the acute abdomen in pregnancy. Obstet Gynecol Clin North Am 2007;34:389–402, x.

Ultrasound for Obstetric Emergencies

Sherelle L. Laifer-Narin, MD[a],*, Nora Tabori, MD[b]

KEYWORDS
• Ultrasound • Obstetric emergencies • Imaging
• Complications

Up to 15% of women will experience a complication during pregnancy. Prompt diagnosis of the problem and appropriate management are imperative to a positive outcome for both the mother and the fetus. Ultrasound is the ideal imaging modality in the pregnant patient because it can be performed at the bedside, is fast, and confers no known risk to the fetus or mother. This article describes the use of ultrasound in the emergent setting. Additional correlative imaging with MRI is presented in difficult cases.

The goal of ultrasound during the first trimester of pregnancy is to confirm a viable intrauterine pregnancy. During the first weeks of gestation, the expected findings will vary depending on the gestational age. Because the findings vary weekly and dating based on last known menstrual period is imprecise, ultrasound findings should also be correlated with β human chorionic gonadotropin (β-hCG) level. In addition to variation with gestational age, the ultrasound technique used (transabdominal vs transvaginal) will result in slight variation in the expected findings at a given stage and therefore must be considered.

The gestational sac is the first widely used definitive finding of pregnancy on ultrasound. The gestational sac is a well-defined, fluid-filled cavity with a hyperechoic rim (Fig. 1). In a normal intrauterine pregnancy, this should be seen eccentrically embedded within the endometrial lining of the body or fundus of the uterus. The gestational sac should be visible by approximately 4 weeks gestation. Although gestational age based on dates can be imprecise, an excellent correlation exists between sac size and β-hCG level.[1]

Although some variation is seen in the accepted range, visualization of a 3-mm gestational sac is expected using transvaginal ultrasound between 1000 and 2000 mIU/mL and transabdominal ultrasound between 2500 and 3600 mIU/mL.[2]

The yolk sac is the first expected structure to be visualized within the gestational sac and confirms viable gestation (Fig. 2). The expected appearance is a round cystic structure with a hyperechoic rim within the gestational sac. The yolk sac is expected to be seen by the fifth week of gestation; in addition, when the gestational sac measures 10 mm, the yolk sac should be visible[3] using both transvaginal and transabdominal techniques.

Shortly after visualization of the yolk sac, the embryo should become visible. The embryo initially appears as a hyperechoic linear structure adjacent to the yolk sac. By the time the gestational sac measures 18 mm, the embryo should always be visible by transvaginal ultrasound. According to Levi and colleagues,[4] embryonic cardiac activity is expected by a crown rump length of 4 mm. Initially, the rate should measure 100 to 115 beats per minute, increasing to 140 beats per minute by the ninth week of gestation. M-mode is the appropriate technique for documenting cardiac activity.

Although the amniotic sac is formed during the fourth week of gestation, it is so closely opposed to the embryo that it may not be visible until more than 7 weeks gestation.

SPONTANEOUS ABORTION

A spontaneous abortion is defined as the spontaneous loss of a conceptus before the 20th week of

[a] Columbia University Medical Center, New York Presbyterian Hospital, 622 West 168th Street, New York, NY 10032, USA
[b] Columbia University NY Presbyterian Medical Center, PGY3 Diagnostic Radiology, 622 West 168th Street, New York, NY 10032, USA
* Corresponding author.
E-mail address: sherellemd@gmail.com

Ultrasound Clin 6 (2011) 177–193
doi:10.1016/j.cult.2011.03.008
1556-858X/11/$ – see front matter © 2011 Published by Elsevier Inc.

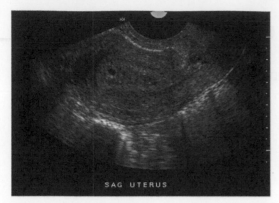

Fig. 1. Early 4-week gestational sac embedded within anterior endometrial wall.

gestation. The rate of spontaneous abortion within the first trimester of pregnancy is estimated to be 15% to 50%, with speculation that the actual rate may be even higher, given that a spontaneous abortion occurring within the first 4 weeks of pregnancy is often not recognized. Genetic abnormalities are present in 80% of all spontaneously aborted pregnancies. Spontaneous abortion has a wide range of risk factors, including advanced maternal age, smoking, advanced paternal age, uterine anomalies, fibroids, infection, iatrogenic, chronic maternal illness, and various pharmaceuticals.[5,6] β-hCG values for patients experiencing a spontaneous abortion range from normal to low.

The five types of abortion are *threatened abortion*, *incomplete abortion*, *missed abortion*, *complete abortion*, and *inevitable abortion* (**Table 1**).

A threatened abortion or threatened miscarriage is a clinical term that refers to vaginal bleeding, abdominal/pelvic pain of any degree, or both during the first 20 weeks of pregnancy. Threatened miscarriage is defined by the absence of passing/passed tissue and a closed internal cervical os. These findings differentiate threatened miscarriage from later stages of miscarriage. Usually the

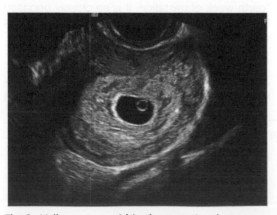

Fig. 2. Yolk sac seen within the gestational sac.

Table 1 Clinical classification of spontaneous abortion	
Type	**Definition**
Threatened abortion	Vaginal bleeding during the first 20 weeks of pregnancy and no evidence of cervical dilation <50% of threatened abortions will progress to loss of pregnancy
Missed abortion	Intrauterine demise of the conceptus without either vaginal bleeding or expulsion of the products of conception
Incomplete abortion	Vaginal bleeding with dilation of the cervix and partial expulsion of the conceptus
Complete abortion	Vaginal bleeding with expulsion of all of the products of conception
Inevitable abortion	Vaginal bleeding with cervical dilation but a maintained intrauterine pregnancy

bleeding is not severe and most of these patients will have a viable embryo or fetus. The ultrasound may show a subchorionic hemorrhage but most will have an otherwise normal early-pregnancy ultrasound examination.

A missed abortion is the failure of an intrauterine pregnancy (IUP) to progress, or the loss of fetal cardiac activity. As set forth by the Royal College of Obstetricians and Gynaecologists, a missed abortion can be definitively diagnosed when a gestational sac larger than 20 mm lacks either an embryo or a yolk sac or there is absence of cardiac activity in an embryo with a crown rump length greater than 5 mm. If neither of these findings is present, a repeat ultrasound should be obtained in 1 week to assess growth; a normal gestational sac increases by approximately 1.1 mm/d; retardation of the growth rate to less than 0.6 mm/d is definitive evidence of an abnormal gestational sac.[7,8]

Differentiation of complete and incomplete abortion is often difficult, and clinical presentation and physical examination may be more definitive. A patient presenting with a complete abortion will report heavy vaginal bleeding, cramping, and passage of tissue that has subsided, whereas a woman presenting with an incomplete abortion has continued heavy bleeding and cramping with or without passage of tissue. In addition, on physical examination a woman with a complete abortion will have blood but no products of conception within the vaginal canal and the cervix will be closed; the patient presenting with an incomplete abortion will have a dilated cervix and products may be seen within either the cervix or the vagina. If retained products of conception are suspected, a classic sonographic finding is the presence of a heterogeneous, mixed echogenic intrauterine mass showing increased vascularity (**Fig. 3**). Blood clots, however, should have an irregular shape with mixed echogenicity and be mobile when compression is applied. If the two cannot be readily differentiated on initial physical examination and ultrasound, observation and short-interval repeat ultrasound are recommended.

The ultrasound findings of an inevitable abortion are more straightforward. Again, the expected findings for gestational age are seen within the uterus, but the cervix will be dilated. Often the products of conception are located within the lower uterine segment or even the cervix.

ECTOPIC PREGNANCY

Ruptured ectopic pregnancy is the leading cause of maternal deaths in the first trimester and accounts for 10% to 15% of all maternal deaths. The incidence has risen from 4.5 to 19.7 cases per 1000 pregnancies from 1970 to 1992. Although increases in certain risk factors have been seen, this is mostly attributed to improved diagnosis.[9]

Ectopic pregnancy is defined as a fertilized egg that implants outside of the uterine cavity. Early recognition of this situation is imperative, because these women have a significant risk for hemorrhage, future infertility, and death. Ectopic implantation occurs in 1% to 2% of all pregnancies. Risk factors include history of ectopic pregnancy, pelvic inflammatory disease (prior or current), tubal ligation/instrumentation, use of an intrauterine device, fertility treatments, smoking, advanced maternal age, salpingitis isthmica nodosum, and prior abdominal surgery, although most cases have no identifiable cause.[10,11]

The most common site of ectopic implantation is the fallopian tube, accounting for approximately 98% of cases. Fallopian tube sites include the ampullary, isthmic, fimbrial, and interstitial portions. Additional sites include the cervix, ovary, cesarean scar, and abdominal cavity. Ultrasound is

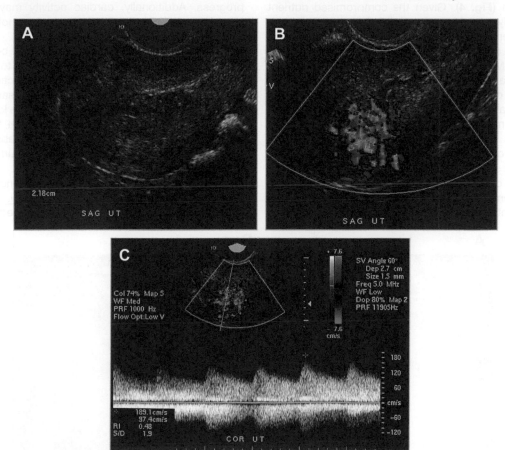

Fig. 3. (*A–C*) Retained products of conception. Intrauterine heterogeneous, mixed echogenic mass with marked internal vascularity in a patient who recently underwent spontaneous abortion.

the most important tool in diagnosing ectopic pregnancy. In patients presenting with abdominal pain with or without vaginal bleeding and a β-hCG of 1500 or more, visualization of an intrauterine gestational sac with or without additional embryonic structures on transvaginal ultrasound is sufficient to exclude ectopic pregnancy. The notable exception to this rule are women undergoing fertility treatment, because they have a significantly higher incidence of heterotopic pregnancy.[12]

A gestational sac is a fluid-filled structure with a hyperechoic rim located eccentrically within one wall of the endometrial lining. Clear visualization of the typical features of a gestational sac is important, because a pseudosac, defined as a collection of fluid within the endometrial cavity secondary to bleeding from the decidualized endometrium, may be seen with an extrauterine pregnancy.

Sonographic evidence of an extrauterine pregnancy is definitive for the diagnosis of an ectopic pregnancy but occurs in fewer than one-third of patients.[13] The appearance of an ectopic conceptus varies widely. In some cases, a normal gestational sac and embryonic structures are visualized (**Fig. 4**). Given the compromised nutrient supply available in the ectopic location, the developmental stage of the conceptus may be delayed when compared with an IUP of comparable gestation. Most commonly the ectopic conceptus will appear as a complex adnexal mass, and is the most common finding of a tubal pregnancy.[14] The appearance of these masses is variable, ranging from mostly cystic to entirely solid. Mobility of the mass independent of the ovary is important for distinction from an ovarian mass.[15] Occasionally, these structures can be confused with a corpus luteum cyst. Characteristically, a corpus luteum has a thinner, less echogenic wall and should not have any internal echoes within the cavity.

The adnexal ring sign corresponding to a hyperechoic, hypervascular ring surrounding an extrauterine gestational sac is the second most common sign of a tubal ectopic pregnancy. Additional extrauterine findings of tubal pregnancies include hematosalpinx, hemoperitoneum, and free pelvic fluid.[16]

Interstitial pregnancies are those that implant within the portion of the proximal fallopian tube just beyond the cavity but are still surrounded by myometrium, and account for 2% to 4% ectopic pregnancies. An eccentrically, superiorly located gestational sac near the uterine fundus with a thin myometrial mantle less than 5 mm suggests a interstitial pregnancy (**Fig. 5**). The echogenic line extending to the uterine horn and bordering the margin of the gestational sac in the intramural portion of the uterus is most specific for interstitial pregnancy and is known as the *interstitial line sign*.[17]

Cervical pregnancy is one that implants within the cervix, and is potentially lethal because of the risk for life-threatening hemorrhage. The gestational sac is round or ovoid, not irregular in shape, thereby allowing differentiation from an abortion in progress. Additionally, cardiac activity may be seen in a cervical pregnancy but would not be seen in an abortion in progress.

Cesarean scar ectopic pregnancies are being reported with increased frequency owing to the increased incidence of prior cesarean sections. Implantation occurs at the site of a prior cesarean section incision, in the anterior portion of the lower uterine segment, at a slightly higher level than a cervical pregnancy. Myometrium is absent between the gestational sac and the urinary bladder (**Fig. 6**).[18]

Even rarer forms of ectopic pregnancies include ovarian pregnancy, abdominal pregnancy, and pregnancies occurring in an anomalous uterine horn.

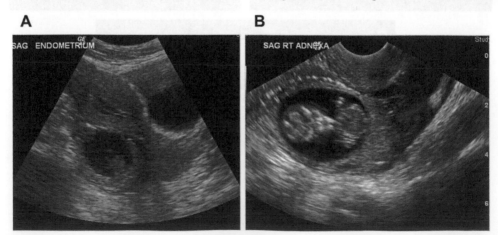

A   **B**

Fig. 4. (*A, B*) Live right tubal ectopic pregnancy. Transabdominal and transvaginal images show empty endometrial cavity, extrauterine gestation in right adnexa with cardiac activity, and free fluid in cul-de-sac.

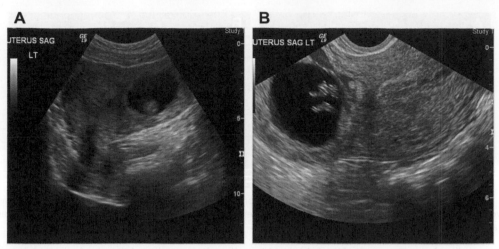

Fig. 5. (*A, B*) Left cornual ectopic pregnancy. Transabdominal and transvaginal images show eccentric, superiorly located gestational sac containing an embryo, near uterine fundus, with a thin myometrial mantle. Note echogenic line from the endometrial cavity to the corner next to the gestational sac.

Criteria for ovarian ectopic pregnancy were established in 1878 by Spiegelberg[19] to confirm that a pregnancy arose in the ovary and did not involve the fallopian tube. Histologic diagnosis is usually necessary to differentiate a true ovarian pregnancy from the much more common tubal ectopic pregnancy (**Fig. 7**). The rise in ovarian pregnancies has been attributed to increased use of intrauterine contraceptive devices, which prevents intrauterine implantation but not ectopic implantation.[20]

In intra-abdominal pregnancies, implantation occurs within the peritoneal cavity. No surrounding myometrium is present, and blood supply is obtained from the omentum and abdominal organs.

Rarely, pregnancy may occur in an anomalous uterus. An entity known as *rudimentary horn pregnancy* occurs in the noncommunicating rudimentary horn associated with a unicornuate uterus. This malformation occurs through transperitoneal migration of spermatozoa through the contralateral tube, with a proposed incidence of 1 in 76,000 to 1 in 140,000 pregnancies. Because rudimentary horn pregnancy results in rupture of the horn and life-threatening hemorrhage during the second or third trimester, early diagnosis is imperative. Ultrasound findings include abnormal appearance of the uterus, suggesting anomalous development, absent continuity of the gestational sac with the uterine cervix, and myometrial tissue completely surrounding the gestational sac. MRI has been useful in clearly delineating these findings (**Fig. 8**).[21]

Given the risk of mortality with rupture, evaluation for free fluid is a key component in examining this patient population. Although a small amount of fluid in the pouch of Douglas is a normal physiologic finding, anechoic free fluid tracking more than one-third of the way up the posterior wall of the

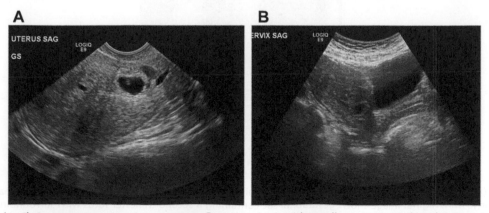

Fig. 6. (*A, B*) Cesarean scar ectopic pregnancy. Gestational sac with a yolk sac implanted at the site of a prior cesarean section incision; no myometrium is visualized.

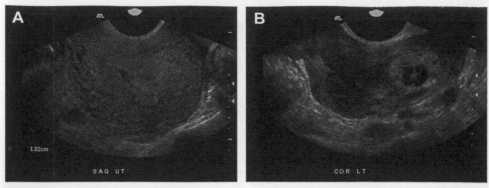

Fig. 7. (A, B) Left ovarian ectopic pregnancy. Empty endometrial cavity, hemoperitoneum, gestational sac with an embryo implanted in the left ovary, pathologically proven. Note ovarian cortex and follicles surrounding ectopic pregnancy.

uterus or a complex appearance of the fluid should increase the suspicion of ectopic pregnancy.[22]

SUBCHORIONIC HEMORRHAGE

A subchorionic hemorrhage or hematoma is defined as a collection of blood products between the uterine wall and the chorionic membrane and may leak through the cervical canal. The risk for miscarriage after subchorionic hemorrhage increases with increasing size and maternal age. Younger gestational age also confers an increased risk of spontaneous abortion. Sonographically,

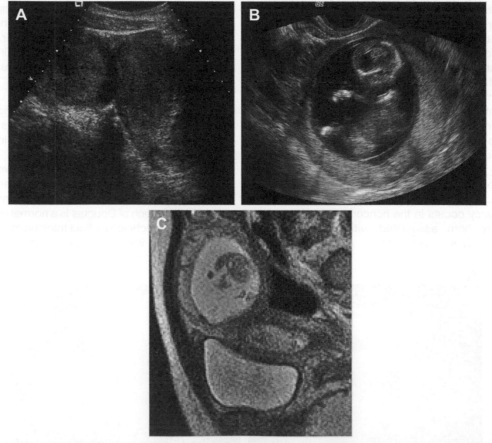

Fig. 8. (A–C) Rudimentary horn pregnancy. Transabdominal image shows empty uterus, with suspicious mass seen superiorly. Transvaginal image shows gestational sac containing a second trimester fetus with surrounding myometrial tissue, consistent with gestation in a noncommunicating rudimentary horn. Sagittal MRI image shows noncommunicating rudimentary horn with surrounding myometrium, superior to unicornuate uterus.

acute hemorrhage appears isoechoic to hypere-choic compared with the chorion, whereas subacute and chronic hemorrhage will appear iso-echoic to hypoechoic (**Fig. 9**).[23]

UTERINE FIBROIDS

Uterine leiomyomas, also known as fibroids, are benign tumors that arise from the overgrowth of smooth muscle and connective tissue in the uterus. Although fibroids are not caused by pregnancy, the incidence of concomitant pregnancy and fibroids is increasing with the use of in vitro fertilization and advanced maternal age. Although the exact mechanism through which fibroids interfere with normal gestation is still unknown, they are associated with multiple obstetrical complications, including preterm labor and spontaneous abortion, and therefore their recognition is important in the management of these patients (**Fig. 10**).[24]

Uterine fibroids are classified based on their location in the uterus and include intramural, submucosal, and subserosal, with intramural the most common. The sonographic appearance of all three types is similar. Typically a heterogeneous, hypoechoic mass with an echogenic rim is seen, although the degree of echogenicity can vary greatly depending on the amount of calcification and fibrous tissue present. During pregnancy, the size and appearance of uterine fibroids may change; this most commonly occurs during the second and third trimesters.[17]

GESTATIONAL TROPHOBLASTIC DISEASES

Gestational trophoblastic disease (GTD) is a spectrum of diseases defined as the abnormal

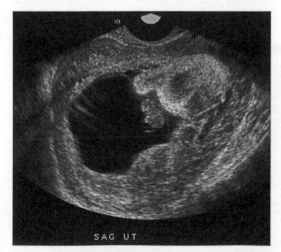

Fig. 9. Acute, hyperechoic subchorionic hemorrhage in a 9-week intrauterine gestation with concomitant fetal demise.

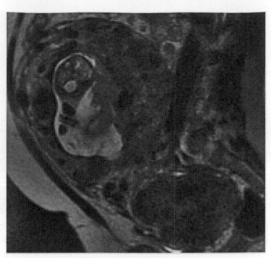

Fig. 10. Large leiomyoma. Sagittal image of the gravid uterus shows innumerable small, predominantly intramural fibroids, with a large dominant fibroid occupying the lower uterine segment and cervix. Patient scheduled for cesarean section.

proliferation of trophoblastic tissue in pregnant or recently pregnant women. GTD can be benign or malignant and is classified into four categories: hydatidiform mole (complete and partial), invasive mole, choriocarcinoma, and placental site trophoblastic tumor.

Initially, GTD manifests with the same signs of early pregnancy; however, as the disease progresses, the β-hCG level rises significantly above the normal levels of pregnancy and the patient often experiences nausea, vomiting, abdominal pain, or vaginal bleeding. Classic findings for complete hydatidiform mole include a uterus that is too large for dating and an intrauterine solid, echogenic mass containing multiple cysts instead of a fetus (**Fig. 11**). In a partial hydatidiform mole, the placenta is enlarged with multiple cystic spaces, and a growth-retarded triploid fetus is present, often with multiple anomalies.

Although marked elevation in the β-hCG and the described classical ultrasound appearance may suggest a diagnosis of molar pregnancy, evacuation and pathologic evaluation are required for definitive diagnosis. If the β-hCG level does not normalize after evacuation within 10 weeks, the disease is classified as persistent or malignant trophoblastic neoplasia.

Invasive mole is characterized by trophoblastic overgrowth and penetration deep into the myometrium, with occasional local invasion, but metastasis is rare (**Fig. 12**). Choriocarcinoma is carcinoma of the chorionic epithelium, and is characterized by trophoblast proliferation, blood vessel erosion, and hematogenous spread of

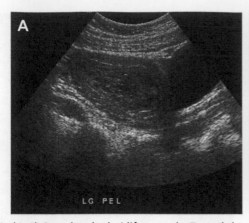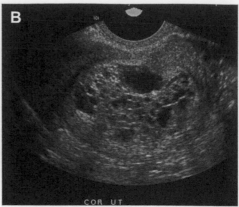

Fig. 11. (A, B) Complete hydatidiform mole. Transabdominal and transvaginal images show a multicystic mass expanding the uterine cavity; no intrauterine gestation is identified.

metastases, most commonly to the lung and vagina, although it can occur anywhere.[25]

Placental site trophoblastic tumor is the rarest form of malignant trophoblastic neoplasia, and is characterized by neoplastic proliferation of intermediate trophoblasts with myometrial invasion at the site of prior placental implantation. Development may occur after a normal pregnancy, ectopic or molar pregnancy, spontaneous abortion, or termination of pregnancy, with the patient presenting with abnormal vaginal bleeding.[26]

OVARIAN HYPERSTIMULATION SYNDROME

Increasingly, patients are undergoing assisted reproductive technology for a variety of reasons. In the setting of assisted reproductive technology, a patient may present with signs and symptoms initially suspicious for ectopic pregnancy. Patients undergoing ovulation induction may develop multiple complications, including third-space

accumulation of fluid, hemoconcentration, renal failure, and thromboembolism. These patients may present with abdominal distension, vomiting, diarrhea, and ascites, and are at increased risk for ovarian torsion, ovarian rupture with hemorrhage, ectopic pregnancy, and infection. Classic ultrasound findings include massive ovarian enlargement with numerous large dominant follicles/cysts, some of which may contain hemorrhagic debris, and ascites.[27]

SECOND TRIMESTER PREGNANCY

The goal of routine second trimester ultrasound is to confirm gestational and assess fetal anatomy, placental implantation, and the amniotic fluid. When considering optimal timing for the anatomy scan, one must consider the earliest point in gestation that the necessary measurements can be achieved and the latest gestation at which an acceptable range of options can be offered to the

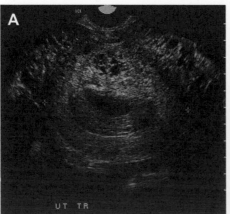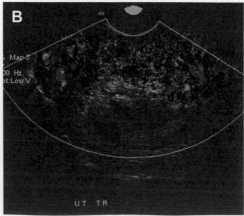

Fig. 12. (A, B) Invasive mole. Transvaginal grayscale and color Doppler imaging show anterior myometrial invasion of gestational trophoblastic disease after dilation and curettage for molar pregnancy.

mother if an abnormality is discovered. Although the details of the second trimester anatomic scan are not discussed here, knowledge of the normal anatomic structures is imperative to understanding of the possible complications that can arise.

PLACENTA PREVIA

Placenta previa is defined as the presence of placental tissue in the lower uterine segment, either partially or completely covering the internal cervical os. Although the exact cause is unknown, the development of placenta previa is believed to result from the implantation of the fertilized ovum into the lower uterine segment. Risk factors for placenta previa include prior placenta previa, prior cesarean delivery, increased maternal age, large placentae, and a maternal history of smoking.[28] The incidence is reported in 1 in 200 to 250 pregnancies. The potential complications include hemorrhage and placental abruption. Although the incidence is relatively high and the complications are potentially life-threatening to both mother and fetus, previa is generally managed expectantly with increased sonographic monitoring, because the conversion rate to normal placental position is nearly 90% between the first and second trimester.[29,30] The migration of the placenta is believed to occur secondary to the rapid growth of the lower uterine segment during the third trimester, resulting in spatial separation of the placenta and the cervix.

If the placenta remains implanted on the cervix, the thinning of the lower uterine segment during late pregnancy can result in various amounts of placental detachment and maternal hemorrhage. The heralding event generally resolves spontaneously without harm to either mother or fetus. There is often no inciting event. During labor, significant fetal hemorrhage also may occur as a result of disrupted villous placental vessels and cesarean section may be necessary.

Traditionally, transabdominal ultrasound was exclusively used to evaluate for placenta previa; however, a study by Timor-Tritsch and Yunis[31] showed that the angle between the probe and cervix allows for safe evaluation without inadvertent entrance into the cervix, which could potentially initiate or worsen bleeding. Sonographically, placenta previa appears as a normal placenta extending down to the level of the cervix with varying degrees of coverage.

PLACENTAL ABRUPTION

Placental abruption is defined as separation of the placenta from the uterine wall after the 20th week of gestation and before birth. It occurs in fewer than 1% of all pregnancies and can result in preterm labor, fetal death, and life-threatening maternal hemorrhage and coagulopathies.[32] Although most cases have no definable cause, risk factors include maternal hypertension, trauma, cigarette smoking, alcohol use, cocaine use, advanced maternal age, abnormal umbilical cord length, amniocentesis, rapid decompression of the uterus from premature rupture of membranes or delivery of the fetus in a multigestational pregnancy, and retroplacental fibroids.[33,34]

Placental abruption is caused by bleeding into the decidua basalis, forcing separation of the placenta from the uterine wall. This complication can cause compression of these structures and compromise of blood supply to the fetus. In some cases, blood can penetrate through the thickness of the uterine wall into the peritoneal cavity, known as *Couvelaire uterus*. Weakening of the myometrium adjacent to the hematoma can result in rupture during contractions, resulting in maternal hemorrhage.

Placental abruption is a clinical diagnosis based on severe abdominal pain, bleeding, and contractions with or without signs of fetal distress at presentation. Although ultrasound has been shown to have a 100% positive predictive value when a retroplacental hematoma is noted, positive findings are only present in 25% of cases and therefore ultrasound is not relied on in this clinical setting.[35] Positive sonographic evidence of abruption is visualization of a heterogeneous retroplacental mass compatible with a blood clot.

VELAMENTOUS INSERTION AND VASA PREVIA

Velamentous insertion is defined as insertion of the umbilical cord into the chorion away from the placental edge, causing the vessels to cross the surface of the membranes to pass into the placenta. The incidence of velamentous insertion is approximately 1% in singleton gestations, but 15% or greater in monozygotic twin pregnancies.[36] Nomiyama and colleagues[37] reported that ultrasound diagnosis of velamentous insertion had a sensitivity and specificity of 100% and 99.8%, respectively.

Vasa previa occurs in the presence of a velamentous cord insertion over the internal cervical os (**Fig. 13**). This complication can result in disruption of the vessels secondary to rupture of the membranes, resulting in fetal hemorrhage and often death. The incidence of vasa previa is 1 in 2000 to 3000 pregnancies. The risk factors include multiple pregnancy, in vitro fertilization, succenturiate lobe or bilobed placenta, and most

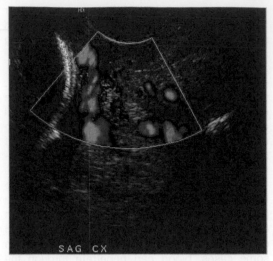

Fig. 13. Vasa previa. Velamentous umbilical vessels are traversing the fetal membranes below the level of the fetal head and crossing the internal os.

significantly a low-lying placenta diagnosed during the second trimester regardless of the position of the placenta at delivery.[38] The outcome of the vasa previa is almost entirely dependent on antenatal diagnosis through ultrasound.

Sonographically, grayscale images will show a series of linear hyperechoic structures crossing the cervical os. Color Doppler studies will show that these are vessels crossing the cervical os.

UTERINE RUPTURE

Uterine rupture is defined as a full-thickness separation of the uterine wall and the overlying serosa. Although the overall incidence is reported at approximately 1 in 1500, a study by Gardeil and colleagues[39] showed that the risk in an unscarred uterus is only approximately 1 in 30,000. The most common causes of scarring include previous cesarean section and myomectomy. Risk factors in the unscarred uterus include multiparity of five or greater, neglected labor, malpresentation, breech extraction, uterine configuration, uterine instrumentation, and most importantly augmentation of labor. Uterine rupture can result in hemorrhage or death in fetus and mother. A study by Leung and colleagues[40] shows that fetal morbidity increases when greater than 18 minutes elapses between the onset of symptoms and delivery.

The initial signs of uterine rupture are often variable. Studies conducted on the clinical indicators of uterine rupture have shown that abnormalities in the fetal heart rate, most notably prolonged deceleration, are the only indicator in 80% to 87% of cases.[41] Sudden maternal abdominal pain is another symptom often described in uterine

rupture, but the reported occurrence is widely variable, ranging from 13% to 60%.

Given the short interval available for the prevention of morbidity and mortality, several studies have been conducted on screening. Rozenberg and colleagues[42] determined that the risk of uterine rupture after previous cesarean delivery was directly related to the thickness of the lower uterine segment during weeks 36 through 38 of gestation, with a 3.5-mm thickness being the threshold of risk. Although the positive predictive value was only 11.8%, the negative predictive value was 99.3%. Another study showed that a wall thickness of 2 mm or less observed within 1 week of delivery had positive and negative predictive values of 73.9% and 100%, respectively.[43] In the acute setting, sonographic findings may include free fluid in the pelvis, and fetal parts, umbilical cord, or placenta external to the uterine cavity.

Uterine rupture is important to distinguish from uterine scar dehiscence. Uterine scar dehiscence is defined as separation of a preexisting scar that does not disrupt the overlying uterine serosa or result in significant bleeding (**Fig. 14**). The integrity of the myometrial wall is breached in uterine rupture (**Fig. 15**).

ABNORMAL PLACENTATION

Abnormal placentation is defined as abnormal adherence of the chorionic villi to the uterine wall and can be classified into three categories (**Table 2**). Life-threatening hemorrhage can result from failure of the placenta to detach from the uterine wall after delivery.

The two most important risk factors for abnormal placentation are prior cesarean section and placenta previa. The causative factor is thought to be a defect of the decidua basalis at the site of the cesarean scar, allowing chorionic villus invasion of the myometrium. Massive hemorrhage can occur at placental separation, with resultant disseminated intravascular coagulation, acute respiratory distress syndrome, renal failure, and death.

Sonographically, these varying degrees of invasion cannot always be readily distinguished, and therefore they are described together. Normally, the decidua basalis can be visualized as a hypoechoic rim between the placenta and the myometrium; progressive loss of this structure (termed the *retroplacental clear space*) is highly suggestive of placenta accreta (**Fig. 16**). Furthermore, multiple hypoechoic regions can be seen within the myometrium, caused by dilated vessels extending from the placenta into the myometrium; this is classically referred to as the *Swiss cheese*

A   B

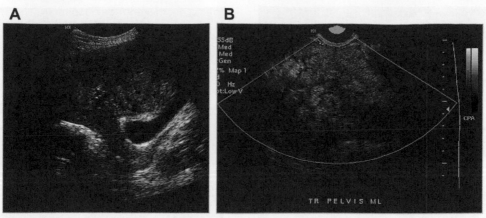

Fig. 14. (*A, B*) Uterine dehiscence. Anterior uterine wall not visible; large heterogeneous mass without internal vascularity consistent with uterine hematoma.

appearance. Doppler analysis of these structures should show turbulent flow. A study by Lerner and colleagues[44] showed that these finding have a sensitivity and specificity of 100% and 94%, respectively.

MRI evaluation of abnormal placentation has become increasingly more common. Useful findings on single-shot fast spin-echo T2-weighted images include contour bulging of the uterus, heterogeneous signal intensity of the placenta,[45] and focal interruption/loss of the hypointense myometrial margin. This latter finding is most helpful in diagnosing placenta percreta in the parametrial regions.[46]

PRETERM LABOR

For a vaginal delivery to occur, the cervix must shorten and dilate. Changes in the cervix are well

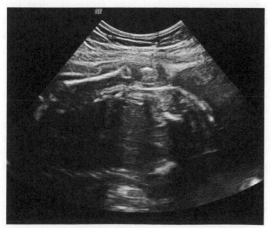

Fig. 15. Uterine rupture. Fetal extremity seen without surrounding myometrium.

visualized with ultrasound, and include cervical shortening and funneling. Prediction of preterm delivery depends on multiple factors, but in all populations, the shorter the cervical length and an earlier time of detection correlate with a higher incidence of preterm delivery (**Fig. 17**).[47]

NONOBSTETRIC EMERGENCIES

Although initial evaluation of a pregnant woman presenting with abdominal pain, fever, bleeding, and various other symptoms will be obstetric, medical and surgical causes for presentation must also be considered. Given the concern for radiation exposure to the fetus, ultrasound is often used for evaluating multiple organs during pregnancy. MRI has been increasingly used to evaluate pregnant patients, owing to the absence of ionizing radiation, multiplanar capability with a wide field of view, and excellent tissue characterization.[48]

GASTROINTESTINAL

The most common nonobstetric surgical emergency in the pregnant patient is acute appendicitis.[49] The appendix is a blind-ending

Table 2		
Classification of abnormal placentation		
Type	**Description**	
Accreta	Chorionic villus attachment to the myometrium	
Increta	Chorionic villus invasion of the myometrium	
Percreta	Chorionic villus invasion through the myometrium and serosa	

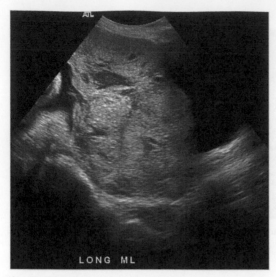

Fig. 16. Placenta accreta/increta/percreta. Transabdominal longitudinal image shows abnormal heterogeneous placenta with hypoechoic regions and loss of myometrial border at the urinary bladder interface consistent with placental invasion.

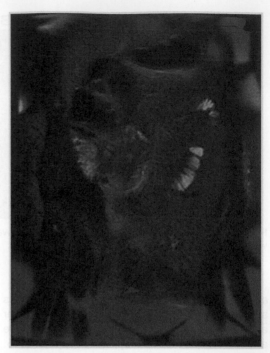

Fig. 18. Acute appendicitis. Single-shot fast spin-echo fat saturation images show periappendiceal fluid surrounding a dilated, blind-ending, tubular structure in a pregnant patient with a 6-week intrauterine pregnancy.

loop of bowel that extends off of the cecum; it generally originates near the ileocecal valve. Acute appendicitis is defined as inflammation of the appendix and is most often caused by blockage of the lumen. In the pregnant patient, presentation of appendicitis may be confusing, because normal anatomy can be distorted by the gravid uterus. MRI can be extremely useful in depicting a dilated appendix, periappendiceal fluid, an appendicolith, or phlegmon for diagnosing appendicitis (**Fig. 18**). Alternatively, a normal appendix excludes appendicitis.

The diagnosis of inflammatory bowel disease during pregnancy is challenging, because symptoms may mimic those that occur during normal pregnancy. MRI can depict dilated bowel loops, bowel obstruction, bowel wall thickening, masses, and abnormal collections (**Figs. 19** and **20**).

HEPATOBILIARY

HELLP syndrome is defined as the triad of hemolytic anemia, elevated liver enzymes, and low platelet count in pregnancy. Patients present with severe right upper quadrant pain and progressive nausea and vomiting. HELLP syndrome has no definite sonographic findings, although hepatomegaly, patchy areas of increased echogenicity, and liver capsule hematoma can occur in some cases.

Gallstones and gallbladder inflammation are well depicted on ultrasound; however, stones within the ductal system are more difficult to identify. MR cholangiopancreatography can be useful for detecting choledocholithiasis (**Fig. 21**).

GENITOURINARY

Both parenchymal and ureteral stones should be considered in pregnant women who present with

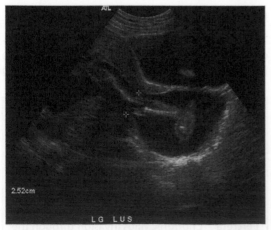

Fig. 17. Preterm labor. Dilated cervix, with fetal parts (foot) presenting in the cervix.

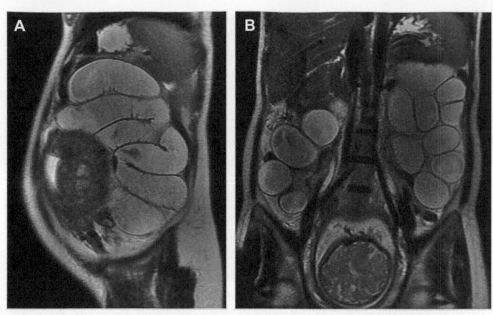

Fig. 19. (*A, B*) Small bowel obstruction. Multiple fluid-filled dilated loops of small bowel.

flank pain and either microscopic or macroscopic blood in the urine. Hydronephrosis is seen in more than 50% of pregnant patients in the third trimester, is secondary to compression of the ureter between the psoas muscle and the gravid uterus, and is termed *physiologic hydronephrosis* (**Fig. 22**). Pathologic hydronephrosis is suspected when the hydronephrosis terminates proximal to the sacral promontory or extends distally, and may be secondary to ureteral calculi, tumor, or blood clots.[49]

GYNECOLOGIC

Abdominal/pelvic pain during pregnancy may be from uterine or ovarian processes. Adnexal masses include nonneoplastic cysts, benign neoplasms, and malignant neoplasms. Adnexal cysts are usually asymptomatic, but may torse and cause exquisite pain (**Fig. 23**). Leiomyomas may be symptomatic during pregnancy secondary to rapid growth, degeneration, or torsion. MRI is

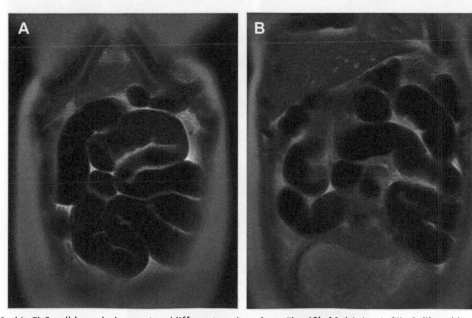

Fig. 20. (*A, B*) Small bowel obstruction (different patient from **Fig. 19**). Multiple air-filled dilated loops of small bowel.

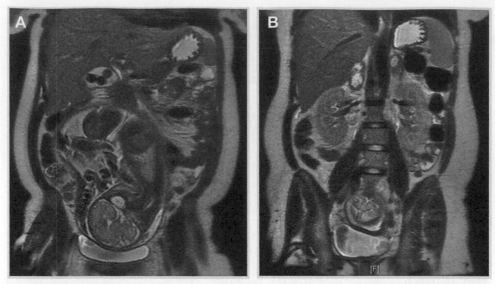

Fig. 21. (*A, B*) Cholelithiasis, bilateral adrenal hemorrhage. Pregnant patient with diffuse abdominal pain; cholelithiasis shown on ultrasound; bilateral adrenal masses consistent with adrenal hemorrhage detected on MRI.

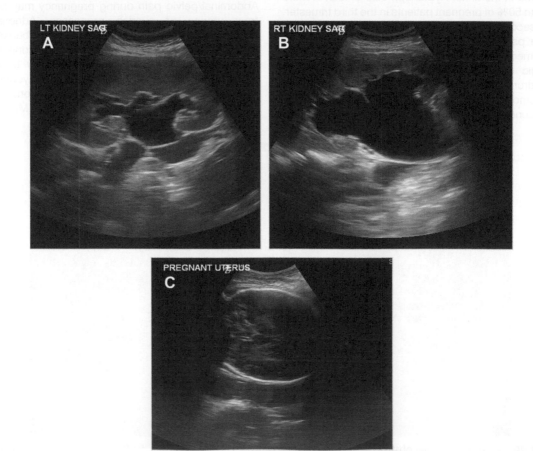

Fig. 22. (*A–C*) Bilateral hydronephrosis of pregnancy, right greater than left.

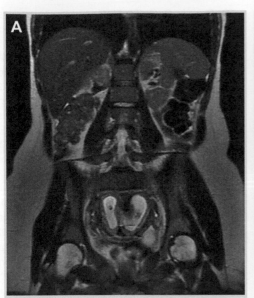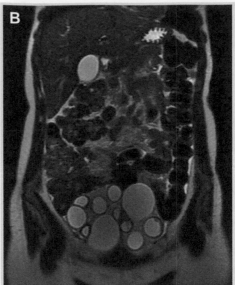

Fig. 23. (*A, B*) Bicornuate uterus, twin gestation, hyperstimulated ovaries. In vitro fertilization patient with abdominal pain. Intrauterine pregnancy seen in each uterine horn; bilateral hyperstimulated ovaries; exploratory laparotomy revealed right adnexal torsion.

extremely useful for diagnosing abdominal/pelvic pain in pregnant patients, especially in the second and third trimester, when the gravid uterus may obscure ultrasound evaluation in the region of pain, and should be used as an adjunct to ultrasound when necessary.

MISCELLANEOUS

Cancer in pregnancy is infrequent, with an estimated incidence of 1 to 2 per 1000 pregnancies. Because complaints of symptoms are often attributable to the pregnancy, the index of suspicion for malignancy by both the patient and physician is low, leading to misdiagnosis or delayed diagnosis. MRI has been useful in evaluating suspicious or persistent symptoms, owing to the lack of ionizing radiation, and global, multiplanar imaging.[50]

In conclusion, ultrasound remains the primary screening modality for initial evaluation of the obstetric patient, with MRI playing an active adjunct role for providing additional diagnostic information.

REFERENCES

1. Nyberg DA, Hill LM. Normal early intrauterine pregnancy: sonographic evidence and HCG correlation. In: Patterson AS, editor. Transvaginal ultrasound. St Louis (MO): Mosby; 1992. p. 64–85.
2. Paspulati RM, Bhatt S, Nour S. Sonographic evaluation of first-trimester bleeding. Radiol Clin North Am 2004;42:297–314.
3. Levi CS, Lyons EA, Lindsay DJ. Early diagnosis of non-viable pregnancy with transvaginal US. Radiology 1998;167:383–5.
4. Levi CS, Lyons EA, Zheng XH, et al. Endovaginal US: demonstration of cardiac activity in embryos of less than 5.0 mm in crown-rump length. Radiology 1990;176:71–4.
5. Arck PC, Rucke M, Rose M, et al. Early risk factors for miscarriage: a prospective cohort study in pregnant women. Reprod Biomed Online 2008;17(1):101–13.
6. Gracia CR, Sammel MD, Chittams J, et al. Risk factors for spontaneous abortion in early symptomatic first-trimester pregnancies. Obstet Gynecol 2005;106(5 Pt 1):993–9.
7. Chudleigh T, Thilaganathan B. Problems of early pregnancy. In: Obstetric ultrasound: how, why, when. London: Elsevier, Churchill Livingston; 2004. p. 51–62.
8. Royal College of Obstetricians and Gynaecologists. Guidance on ultrasound procedures in early pregnancy. London: RCOG Press; 1995.
9. Tenore JL. Ectopic pregnancy. Am Fam Physician 2000;61(4):1080–8.
10. DeStefano F, Peterson HB, Layde PM, et al. Risk of ectopic pregnancy following tubal sterilization. Obstet Gynecol 1982;60(3):326–30.
11. Diquelou JY, Pia P, Tesquier L, et al. The role of Chlamydia trachomatis in the infectious etiology of extrauterine pregnancy. J Gynecol Obstet Biol Reprod 1988;17(3):325–32 [in French].
12. Dor J, Seidman DS, Levran D, et al. The incidence of combined intrauterine and extrauterine pregnancy

after in vitro fertilization and embryo transfer. Fertil Steril 1991;55(4):833–4.

13. Patel MD. Rule out ectopic: asking the right questions, getting the right answers. Ultrasound Q 2006;22(2):87–100.

14. Frates MC, Brown DL, Doubilet PM, et al. Tubal rupture in patients with ectopic pregnancy: diagnosis with transvaginal US. Radiology 1994;191(3):769–72.

15. Blaivas M. Color Doppler in the diagnosis of ectopic pregnancy in the emergency department: is there anything beyond a mass and fluid? J Emerg Med 2002;22(4):379–84.

16. Lin EP, Bhatt S, Dogra VS. Diagnostic clues to ectopic pregnancy. Radiographics 2008;28(6):1661–71.

17. Ackerman TE, Levi CS, Dashefsky SM, et al. Interstitial line: sonographic finding in interstitial (cornual) ectopic pregnancy. Radiology 1993;189(1):83–7.

18. Levine D. Ectopic pregnancy. Radiology 2007;245(2):385–97.

19. Berek JS, Novak E. Berek and Novak's Gynecolog. 14th edition. New York: Lippincott Williams and Wilkins; 2006. p. 627.

20. Sturm JT, Hankins DG, Malo JW, et al. Ovarian ectopic pregnancy. Ann Emerg Med 1984;13(5):362–4.

21. Tsafrir A, Rojansky N, Sela HY, et al. Rudimentary horn pregnancy: first-trimester prerupture sonographic diagnosis and confirmation by magnetic resonance imaging. J Ultrasound Med 2005;24(2):219–23.

22. Dart R, McLean SA, Dart L. Isolated fluid in the cul-de-sac: how well does it predict ectopic pregnancy? Am J Emerg Med 2002;20(1):1–4.

23. Abu-Yousef MM, Bleicher JJ, Williamson RA, et al. Subchorionic hemorrhage: sonographic diagnosis and clinical significance. AJR Am J Roentgenol 1987;149(4):737–40.

24. Lev-Toaff AS, Coleman BG, Arger PH, et al. Leiomyomas in pregnancy: sonographic study. Radiology 1987;164:375–80.

25. Green CL, Angtuaco TL, Shah HR, et al. Gestational trophoblastic disease: a spectrum of radiologic diagnosis. Radiographics 1996;16(6):1371–84.

26. Allen SD, Lim AK, Seckl MJ, et al. Radiology of gestational trophoblastic neoplasia. Clin Radiol 2006;61(4):301–13.

27. Madill JJ, Mullen NB, Harrison BP. Ovarian hyperstimulation syndrome: a potentially fatal complication of early pregnancy. J Emerg Med 2008;35(3):283–6.

28. Gilliam M, Rosenberg D, Davis F. The likelihood of placenta previa with greater number of cesarean deliveries and higher parity. Obstet Gynecol 2002;99(6):976–80.

29. Mustafa SA, Brizot ML, Carvalho MH. Transvaginal ultrasonography in predicting placenta previa at delivery: a longitudinal study. Ultrasound Obstet Gynecol 2002;20(4):356–9.

30. Rizos N, Doran TA, Miskin M, et al. Natural history of placenta previa ascertained by diagnostic ultrasound. Am J Obstet Gynecol 1979;133:287–91.

31. Timor-Tritsch IE, Yunis RA. Confirming the safety of transvaginal sonography in patients suspected of placenta previa. Obstet Gynecol 1990;81:742–4.

32. Combs CA, Nyberg DA, Mack LS, et al. Expectant management after sonographic diagnosis of placental abruption. Am J Perinatol 1992;9:170–4.

33. Abu-Heija A, al-Chalabi H, el-Iloubani N. Abruptio placentae: risk factors and perinatal outcome. J Obstet Gynaecol Res 1998;24(2):141–4.

34. Hoskins IA, Friedman DM, Frieden FJ. Relationship between antepartum cocaine abuse, abnormal umbilical artery Doppler velocimetry, and placental abruption. Obstet Gynecol 1991;78(2):279–82.

35. Glantz C, Purnell L. Clinical utility of sonography in the diagnosis and treatment of placental abruption. J Ultrasound Med 2002;21:837–40.

36. Lopriore E, Sueters M, Middeldorp JM, et al. Velamentous cord insertion and unequal placental territories in monochorionic twins with and without twin-to-twin-transfusion syndrome. Am J Obstet Gynecol 2007;196:159.e1–5.

37. Nomiyama M, Toyota Y, Kawano H. Antenatal diagnosis of velamentous umbilical cord insertion and vasa previa with color Doppler imaging. Ultrasound Obstet Gynecol 1998;12(6):377–9.

38. Oyelese KO, Turner M, Lees C, et al. Vasa previa: an avoidable obstetric tragedy. Obstet Gynecol Surv 1999;54:138–45.

39. Gardeil F, Daly S, Turner MJ. Uterine rupture in pregnancy reviewed. Eur J Obstet Gynecol Reprod Biol 1994;56(2):107–10.

40. Leung AS, Leung EK, Paul RH. Uterine rupture after previous cesarean delivery: maternal and fetal consequences. Am J Obstet Gynecol 1993;169:945–50.

41. Bujold E, Mehta SH, Bujold C, et al. Interdelivery interval and uterine rupture. Am J Obstet Gynecol 2002;187(5):1199–202.

42. Rozenberg P, Goffinet F, Philippe HJ, et al. Thickness of the lower uterine segment: its influence in the management of patients with previous cesarean sections. Eur J Obstet Gynecol Reprod Biol 1999;87(1):39–45.

43. Gotoh H, Masuzaki H, Yoshida A, et al. Predicting incomplete uterine rupture with vaginal sonography during the late second trimester in women with prior cesarean. Obstet Gynecol 2000;95(4):596–600.

44. Lerner JP, Deane S, Timor-Tritsch IE. Characterization of placenta accrete using transvaginal sonography and color Doppler imaging. Ultrasound Obstet Gynecol 1995;5:198–201.

45. Lax A, Prince MR, Mennitt KW, et al. The value of specific MRI features in the evaluation of suspected placental invasion. Magn Reson Imaging 2007;25(1):87–93.

46. Kim JA, Narra VR. Magnetic resonance imaging with true fast imaging with steady-state precession and half-Fourier acquisition single-shot turbo spin-echo sequences in cases of suspected placenta accreta. Acta Radiol 2004;45(6):692–8.

47. Mella MT, Berghella V. Prediction of preterm birth: cervical sonography. Semin Perinatol 2009;33(5):317–24.

48. Beddy P, Keogan MT, Sala E, et al. Magnetic resonance imaging for the evaluation of acute abdominal pain in pregnancy. Semin Ultrasound CT MR 2010; 31(5):433–41.

49. Brown MA, Birchard KR, Semelka RC. Magnetic resonance evaluation of pregnant patients with acute abdominal pain. Semin Ultrasound CT MR 2005;26(4):206–11.

50. Moran BJ, Yano H, Al Zahir N, et al. Conflicting priorities in surgical intervention for cancer in pregnancy. Lancet Oncol 2007;8(6):536–44.

Ultrasonographic Evaluation of Acute Urinary Tract and Male Genitourinary Pathology

Ryan J. Smith, MD*, Mindy M. Horrow, MD

KEYWORDS

- Ultrasonography • Emergency • Urinary tract
- Male genitalia

ASSESSMENT OF THE URINARY TRACT

In the emergency setting, computed tomography (CT) is usually the imaging study of choice for evaluation of the kidneys and bladder with respect to calculi, infections, and trauma. However, in certain populations, such as children, young adults, pregnant women, or people with acute exacerbations of chronic disease, a somewhat less sensitive study without ionizing radiations may be more appropriate. Benefits of ultrasonography include portability, relatively low cost, and ability to localize pain in real time. In patients who cannot receive intravenous contrast, the sensitivity of CT decreases for diagnoses such as pyelonephritis or renal vein thrombosis and ultrasonography may become a better alternative. This section discusses the use of ultrasonography for acute flank pain and suspected nephroureterolithiasis, urinary tract infection, trauma, and several miscellaneous applications.

Urinary Tract Calculi and Acute Flank Pain

Although noncontrast CT is the gold standard for the diagnosis of urolithiasis, with sensitivities of 95% to 98% and specificities of 96% to 100%,[1] ultrasonography with modern equipment and techniques may, in certain situations, achieve a similar degree of accuracy. The challenge in performing ultrasonography is to image the entire collecting system, to detect or potentially exclude an obstructing calculus. The intrarenal collecting system, renal pelvis, and urinary bladder are most easily accessed by sonography for the presence of calculi. Although the normal ureter is too small to image with ultrasonography, when dilated because of obstruction it may be more easily visualized unless obscured by overlying bowel gas. The distal ureter can often be imaged using the distended bladder as a sonographic window (Fig. 1).

There are few studies of direct comparison between noncontrast CT and ultrasonography for renal and ureteral calculi. Sheafor and colleagues[2] reported 96% and 61% sensitivities for CT and ultrasonography, respectively, in 23 patients with flank pain who were ultimately diagnosed with ureteral calculi. Park and colleagues[3] reported an ultrasonographic sensitivity of 98% for the detection of ureteral calculi among 296 patients who fasted for 8 hours and received vigorous intravenous hydration to optimize the sonographic exam. Patlas and colleagues[4] reported on 62 patients with suspected renal colic who prospectively underwent both ultrasonography and non–contrast-enhanced CT. Using stone recovery or urological interventions as the gold standard, the sensitivity and specificity of ultrasonography were 93% and 95%, respectively, for the detection of calculi when compared 91% and 95%, respectively, for CT. The ultrasonographic examinations were performed transabdominally after ingestion

Albert Einstein Medical Center, Jefferson Medical College, Philadelphia, PA, USA
* Corresponding author.
E-mail address: smithry@einstein.edu

Ultrasound Clin 6 (2011) 195–213
doi:10.1016/j.cult.2011.03.007
1556-858X/11/$ – see front matter © 2011 Elsevier Inc. All rights reserved.

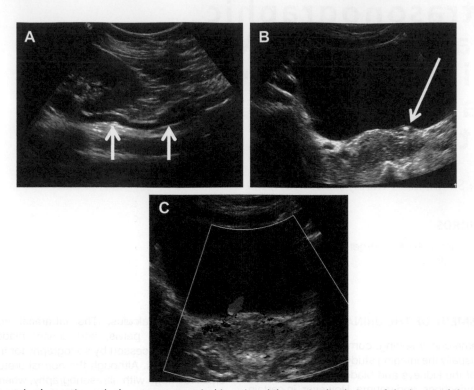

Fig. 1. Acutely obstructing calculus at ureterovesical junction. (*A*) Longitudinal view of the lower of the pole left kidney shows dilated renal pelvis and ureter (*arrows*). (*B*) Transverse view of distended bladder with calculus at left ureteropelvic junction (*arrow*). (*C*) Transverse view of bladder with color Doppler only showed jets from right ureteral orifice.

of 400 mL of water. In addition, ultrasonography detected 6 of 7 alternative diagnoses to explain the patient's pain, only missing 1 case of appendicitis detected by CT. A slightly lower sensitivity of ultrasonography was found in the prospective study of Ripolles and colleagues.[5] In 66 patients, the ultrasonographic sensitivity for ureteral calculi was 79% compared with 93% for CT. Hydration was used when the ureter could not be visualized initially, or the bladder was empty. There were 2 false-negative cases on CT reported as phleboliths that were correctly identified as ureteral calculi on ultrasonography. Direct visualization of a distal ureteral calculus can be significantly improved by using alternative types of scanning. Mitterberger and colleagues[6] found a sensitivity of 55% for distal ureteral calculi using standard transabdominal techniques. The sensitivity improved to 100% by using transrectal imaging in men and transvaginal imaging in women. Median size of the calculi was 4.4 mm.

Urinary tract calculi typically appear as echogenic foci with posterior acoustic shadowing. Renal calculi in kidneys without hydronephrosis may be more difficult to perceive within the echogenic sinus. In addition, posterior shadowing may be weak or absent depending on the composition

and size of the calculus and the amount of attenuating retroperitoneal and renal sinus fat. Depending on the size and extent of shadowing, it can also be difficult to adequately determine the number and size of the calculi on ultrasonography. Posterior shadowing can be accentuated by careful sonographic technique including increased transducer frequency, narrow focal zone, harmonic imaging, and removal of smoothing algorithms. Vascular calcifications can be confounding on both ultrasonography and CT. Other mimics of renal calculi include gas, milk of calcium cysts, cortical and medullary calcifications, a prominent junctional parenchymal line, catheters, and small echogenic tumors.[7]

Theoretically, bladder calculi should be easier to appreciate because they are surrounded by anechoic urine but could be overlooked if the bladder is not well distended. Maneuvers such as rolling the patient into a decubitus position may also be necessary to facilitate identification of stones. Difficulties may be encountered with gas in the bladder, calcified tumors, or stones located in bladder diverticula.

Color and power Doppler twinkling or comet-tail artifacts may improve the sensitivity for calculi. This poorly understood artifact consists of a rapidly changing color signal with aliasing just deep to the object from which it originates. It occurs more commonly at lower frequencies and may be more easily perceived in the kidney by increasing the filter and pulse repetition frequency to decrease the amount of color Doppler signal from adjacent vascular structures. The color twinkle may allow visualization of a ureteral calculus that otherwise would have blended into the retroperitoneal fat. This artifact has great value because it is easy to apply and appreciate. Color twinkling has been reported in 83% to 86% of urinary tract calculi (**Fig. 2**).[8]

It is widely appreciated that the secondary findings of acute urinary tract obstruction on CT can be as sensitive for the diagnosis of renal colic as direct visualization of the obstructing calculus. On sonography, the findings of hydronephrosis, perinephric fluid, renal enlargement, absent or diminished ureteral jets, edema at the ureteral orifice, and an elevation of resistive index may prove helpful when the calculus is not seen. A comparison study found that the sensitivities of CT and ultrasonography improved to 100% and 92%, respectively, by considering relevant secondary findings.[2]

Hydronephrosis is the most easily appreciated secondary finding in patients with an acutely obstructing ureteral calculus. However, it may be absent in up to 19% of patients, especially in the first few hours after obstruction.[4] In addition, there are a variety of findings that may simulate hydronephrosis on sonography. Color Doppler should always be used to distinguish mild hydronephrosis from prominent intrarenal vessels. Occasionally, parapelvic cysts may simulate a dilated collecting system. Whenever hydronephrosis is present, the dilated ureter should be traced distally as far as possible to determine the level and cause of obstruction. The mid portion of the ureter is the most difficult segment to visualize sonographically. Visualization can be improved in some patients by using decubitus positioning and manual compression of bowel gas. Lastly, it is important to remember that dilatation of the collecting system may occur without obstruction in patients presenting with acute urinary tract symptoms, particularly in those with pyelonephritis.

Gray-scale findings other than hydroureteronephrosis are generally more subtle and difficult to appreciate compared with noncontrast CT. Small amounts of perinephric fluid may be present with an acutely obstructing calculus. Larger perinephric collections are likely due to forniceal rupture. Studies of noncontrast CT have shown that the extent of perinephric stranding is related to the duration of symptoms. Renal enlargement may be difficult to appreciate unless marked or if there is a prior examination for comparison. Peristaltic spurts of urine entering the bladder can be visualized on intravenous urography, contrast CT, and ultrasonography. These jets can be appreciated on gray-scale imaging as focal bursts of low-level echoes into otherwise anechoic urine, but recognition of this flow is facilitated by color Doppler imaging. Although the overall frequency of normal ureteral jets is variable even in well-hydrated patients, the frequency and magnitude is comparable from side to side when observed over a few minutes. Thus, fewer, less-exuberant, or continuous jets from 1 ureteral orifice can be used as a secondary sign of obstruction in a patient with ipsilateral flank pain (see **Fig. 1C**).[9]

Over the past 2 decades, many have investigated the utility of spectral Doppler to increase the sensitivity of gray-scale imaging for the assessment of renal dysfunction, including acute obstruction. The resistive index ([peak systole − end diastole]/peak systole) of arcuate or interlobar

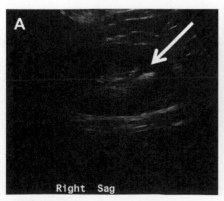
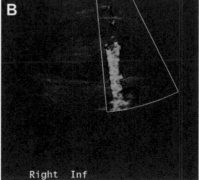

Fig. 2. Twinkle artifact helps confirm lower pole calculus in obese patient. (*A*) Calculus suspected in lower pole as echogenic focus with questionable posterior shadow (*arrow*). (*B*) Color Doppler imaging shows prominent twinkle artifact confirming the calculus.

arteries is the parameter most studied in this regard. Despite the initial promising reports, most investigators have found low sensitivities and specificities for the Doppler diagnosis of acute obstruction. Likely reasons include the common occurrence of partial obstruction and the vasodilatory aspects of nonsteroidal inflammatory drugs commonly used to treat the pain of acute ureteral colic. Since the universal acceptance of noncontrast CT for ureteral calculi, little further research has been done in this area.[10]

In summary, noncontrast CT, especially with low-dose techniques, has become the premier imaging modality for renal colic. Its widespread acceptance by emergency room physicians as the imaging modality of choice has stifled further interest in the use of sonography. Nonetheless, there are some, small promising studies indicating a utility of ultrasonography. Whereas CT will likely continue as the first-line imaging study, ultrasonography should be considered in patients with repeated episodes of ureteral colic and especially in young adults, children, and pregnant patients to reduce the radiation burden. Meticulous ultrasonographic technique is required, including hydration, color Doppler imaging for ureteral jets and twinkle artifacts, and supplementation of transabdominal imaging with transvaginal techniques for distal ureteral calculi.

Urosepsis

Most lower urinary tract infections do not require any diagnostic imaging. Imaging is often performed for suspected upper urinary tract infections, inconclusive diagnoses, and evaluation of superimposed obstruction. Even though CT with intravenous contrast is the most sensitive and rapidly performed emergency study, its utility decreases if intravenous contrast cannot be used because of renal insufficiency and allergic reactions and in renal transplant patients. Ultrasonography can be useful in these situations, as well as in pregnant and younger patients in whom ionizing radiation should be minimized.

Pyelonephritis, especially when mild, usually results in a normal renal sonogram. When abnormalities are noted, diffuse renal enlargement is the most common finding. More subtle parenchymal abnormalities can sometimes be appreciated, especially in thinner patients or with higher-frequency transducers. These abnormalities include subtle ill-defined regions of increased and occasionally decreased echogenicity with loss of corticomedullary differentiation and focal swelling. Color Doppler of these regions show relatively diminished perfusion, corresponding to focal areas of decreased contrast enhancement on CT (Fig. 3).[11,12] Mild pelvocaliectasis and small amounts of perinephric fluid are nonspecific findings. Occasionally, urothelial thickening or gas in the collecting system or parenchyma may be appreciated, although large amounts of parenchymal gas may completely obscure the kidney.

More complex infections can also be detected on ultrasonography. A renal abscess appears as a complex hypoechoic mass, sometimes with through transmission or dependent debris (Fig. 4). The appearance overlaps a variety of renal lesions including hemorrhagic cysts and tumors. A perinephric abscess may develop from rupture of a renal abscess into the perinephric space or from secondary infection of a traumatic or iatrogenic hematoma or urinoma. A perinephric abscess appears as a complex fluid collection in the perinephric space, and because it may spread throughout the retroperitoneum, its full extent is often better appreciated on CT. Pyonephrosis refers to purulent material in an obstructed collecting system. This condition requires emergency

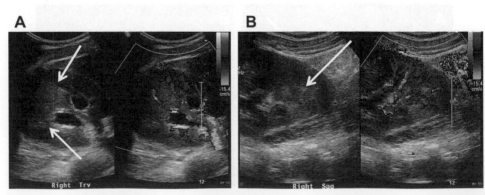

Fig. 3. Acute pyelonephritis. (A) Transverse split screen gray-scale and color compare images show region of slightly increased echogenicity (arrows) with relatively decreased color flow. (B) Longitudinal image shows that the same hyperechoic region (arrow) with decreased flow is in the lower pole.

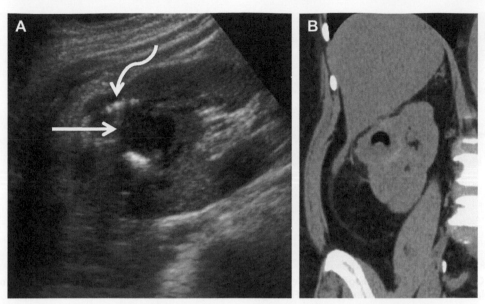

Fig. 4. Renal abscess. (*A*) Transverse image of the upper pole of the right kidney with complex cystic lesions with nondependent bright echoes (*curved arrow*) and dirty posterior shadow characteristic of gas (*white arrow*). (*B*) CT confirms gas-containing abscess.

decompression of the obstructed kidney and carries a significant morbidity and mortality. Ultrasonography often demonstrates internal echoes, gas, or fluid debris levels, even though infected urine may appear anechoic (**Fig. 5**). Because the findings can be subtle, a high index of suspicion is necessary in any patient with urosepsis and hydronephrosis.

Although cystitis does not usually warrant imaging, ultrasonography may show diffuse wall thickening (**Fig. 6**). If the cystitis is focal, or severe with hemorrhagic changes, the appearance may be indistinguishable from that of a tumor. Imaging is often limited because the patient is unable to tolerate adequate distention of the bladder. With emphysematous infections, the gas in the wall or

lumen may completely obscure the bladder. Infected urine often demonstrates low-level echoes on ultrasonography (**Fig. 7**).

In a variety of acute situations, bladder ultrasonography may be helpful. In patients presenting acutely without urine output, ultrasonography can rapidly determine the presence and volume of a distended urinary bladder. It can also be used to guide and check Foley catheter placement and differentiate a cystic pelvic mass from a distended bladder.

Trauma

Evaluation of the kidneys and bladder after blunt or penetrating trauma is almost exclusively the

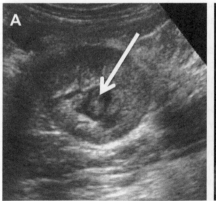
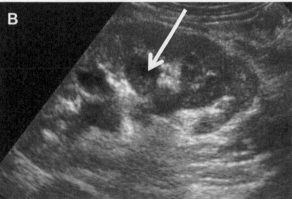

Fig. 5. Pyonephrosis. (*A*) Transverse and (*B*) longitudinal views show dilated calyces filled with dependent echogenic material (*arrows*).

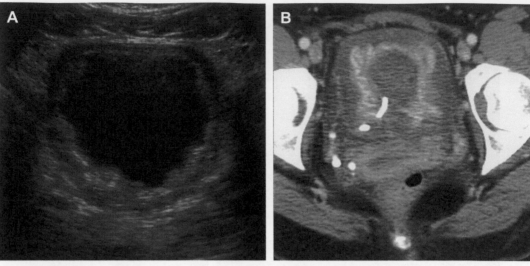

Fig. 6. Cystitis. (*A*) Transverse image of bladder with diffusely thickened wall. (*B*) CT with contrast confirms thickened bladder wall with enhancing mucosa. Findings resolved with treatment.

purview of contrast-enhanced CT, other than the focused assessment with sonography in trauma scan to evaluate for free fluid. Acute perinephric hematomas, even when large, may blend into the renal cortex and be difficult to appreciate. Focal renal hematomas and contusions can be recognized, even though bowel gas and the inability to image from different positions in many trauma patients may limit the sensitivity of sonography to detect renal injury when compared with hepatic and splenic injuries (**Fig. 8**). Ultrasonography is of little use in distinguishing intraperitoneal and extraperitoneal bladder ruptures.[13]

Ultrasonography, particularly with color Doppler may be more useful in the sequelae of iatrogenic renal trauma from renal biopsy, ablation, or catheter placement. Knowing the location of the

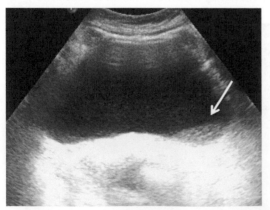

Fig. 7. Bladder filled with infected urine. Transverse view of distended bladder with increased gain shows complex urine with layering of debris (*arrow*).

procedure, one can better evaluate for an expanding hematoma. If obstruction of the collecting system occurs because of intrinsic or extrinsic blood clots, ultrasonography can be used to follow its resolution. Using color Doppler immediately after a procedure allows visualization of acute bleeding with a patent track[14] or a traumatic arteriovenous fistula or pseudoaneurysm (**Fig. 9**).

Acute Vascular Pathology

Ultrasonography can be a primary diagnostic tool in a variety of miscellaneous acute situations. It is particularly useful for the evaluation of vascular abnormalities when contrast cannot be used. Acute global or segmental renal artery occlusion appears entirely normal on gray-scale imaging, but become obvious with color and duplex Doppler imaging. Renal artery embolism should be considered in predisposed patients with cardiac arrhythmias or acute myocardial infarction and acute flank pain especially with hematuria (**Fig. 10**). Acute renal artery thrombosis is more likely after blunt trauma or is secondary to arterial dissection. Ultrasonographic imaging in such patients should always include Doppler.

Acute renal vein thrombosis usually results in the nonspecific findings of an enlarged, hypoechoic kidney with poor corticomedullary differentiation. The acute thrombus may be difficult to appreciate in gray scale, but Doppler imaging shows lack of venous flow and an elevated resistive index, often with reversal of diastolic flow (**Fig. 11**).[15] In addition, ultrasonography can distinguish extrinsic causes of renal vein thrombosis, such as a retroperitoneal mass or lymphadenopathy, and

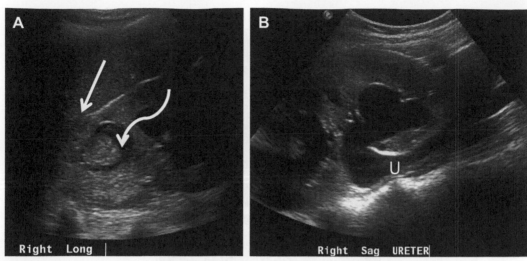

Fig. 8. Pregnant patient presented with hematuria after a motor vehicle accident. (*A*) Longitudinal view of the upper pole of the right kidney with ill-defined hyperechoic region without an intact overlying capsule (*straight arrow*) and calyceal dilatation with blood clot (*curved arrow*). The findings indicate a renal laceration with thrombus, which likely extends to involve the collecting system (*B*) Longitudinal view of the renal pelvis and lower pole with urine blood level in dilated calyx and low-level echoes in dilated ureter (U).

evaluate the inferior vena cava, iliac veins, and other veins for the extent of venous thrombosis (**Fig. 12**). Ultrasonographic contrast agents have shown promise to increase the sensitivity and specificity of this technique for acute vascular and infectious diagnoses and may become useful in the emergency setting if approved for use in this country.[16]

In summary, although CT is the most commonly used imaging modality for the kidneys and bladder in the emergency setting, considerations of contrast and radiation dose warrant the use of ultrasonography as a primary imaging modality in certain situations. Detailed clinical information can guide the sonographer to search for specific diagnoses, using color and spectral Doppler as needed, always with an understanding of the limitations of sonography, particularly in large patients.

ASSESSMENT OF ACUTE MALE GENITOURINARY PATHOLOGY

Ultrasonography, including color and pulsed Doppler imaging, is the primary modality for the evaluation of acute scrotal pain. The objective of ultrasonography is to determine the cause of pain and to differentiate between patients who need to be treated urgently with surgery and those

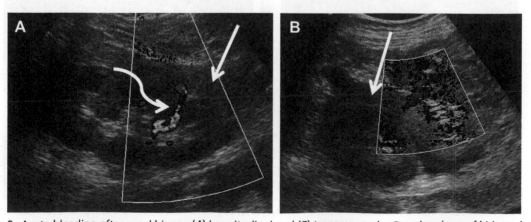

Fig. 9. Acute bleeding after renal biopsy. (*A*) Longitudinal and (*B*) transverse color Doppler views of kidney show acute hemorrhage with adjacent perinephric hematoma (*arrows*) that expanded during real-time imaging. The presence of an arterial jet (*curved arrow, A*) indicates active bleeding.

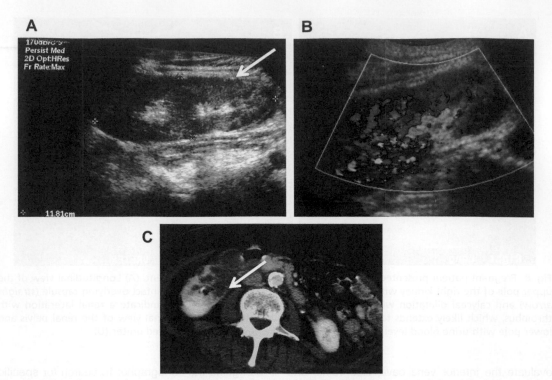

Fig. 10. Infarct lower pole of the right kidney. (*A*) Longitudinal gray-scale image of the right kidney shows slightly increased echogenicity of the lower pole (*arrow*). (*B*) Color Doppler image shows a markedly decreased flow in the lower pole. (*C*) CT with contrast confirms wedge-shaped hypodense region with capsular "rim sign" (*arrow*) characteristic of an infarct.

who should be treated medically. The primary differential considerations, in the setting of acute scrotal pain, include infection, torsion, and trauma. The various causes of acute scrotal pain and their sonographic features are reviewed.

Infection

Epididymitis and orchitis
Color Doppler ultrasonography is the primary imaging modality for the evaluation of scrotal, testicular, and epididymal infections. Epididymitis

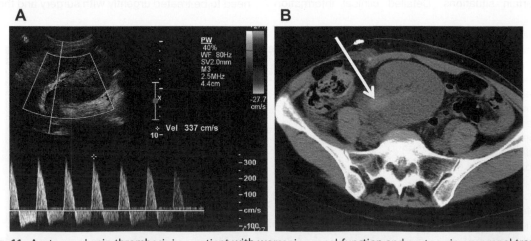

Fig. 11. Acute renal vein thrombosis in a patient with worsening renal function and acute pain over renal transplant. (*A*) Transverse view of the kidney shows only arterial flow with high-resistance waveforms characterized by reversal of flow during diastole and no visible venous flow. (*B*) Corresponding noncontrast CT shows high density in thrombosed renal vein (*arrow*).

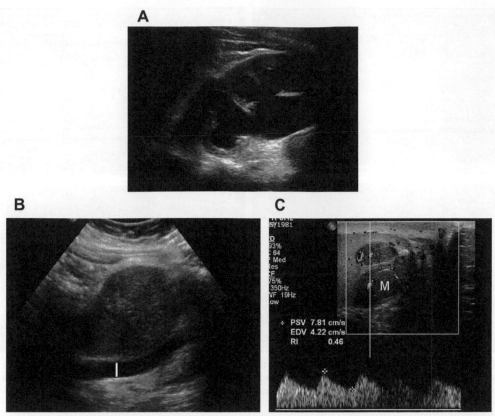

Fig. 12. A 30-year-old man with left flank pain. (*A*) Longitudinal view of the left kidney with severe hydronephrosis. (*B*) Longitudinal view of the inferior cava (I) shows compression by large conglomerate of adenopathy. (*C*) Subsequent imaging of the left testis demonstrates a lobulated hypoechoic mass (M) with low-resistance flow. Seminoma was proved on biopsy.

results most commonly from an ascending urinary tract infection. Sexually transmitted diseases, such as those caused by *Chlamydia trachomatis* and *Neisseria gonorrhoeae*, are most common in young adults, whereas in children and men older than 35 years, the disease is most frequently caused by *Escherichia coli* and *Proteus mirabilis*.[17] Viral and tuberculous infections are less common. The entire epididymis or just a portion, such as the head, body, or tail, can be involved. On gray-scale imaging, the epididymis is enlarged and heterogeneously hypoechoic. On color Doppler imaging, there is increased vascularity throughout the affected portion (**Fig. 13**). In subtle cases, it is important to compare the affected epididymis to the normal side in order to qualitatively appreciate the increase in flow. In chronic or partially treated infection, the epididymis becomes hypoechoic and vascularity becomes normal to relatively decreased. The infection can progress if not fully or properly treated, and an abscess can develop. An abscess appears as a well-circumscribed, avascular complex hypoechoic collection within

the epididymis (**Fig. 14**). Debris or fluid-fluid levels may also be present within an abscess.

Orchitis usually occurs in association with epididymitis. Isolated orchitis is less common but can be seen in the setting of viral infections such as mumps. On gray-scale imaging, the testis is usually enlarged and hypoechoic, whereas color Doppler imaging reveals increased vascularity (**Fig. 15**). Color Doppler analysis is more sensitive in the diagnosis of orchitis than gray-scale imaging alone because hypervascularity may be the only abnormal finding. Horstman and colleagues[18] found hyperemia to be the only sonographic finding of inflammation in 20% of cases of epididymitis and in 40% of cases of orchitis. Focal orchitis can be a more challenging diagnosis because it can appear similar to a testicular mass. Focal orchitis appears as an area of relatively decreased echogenicity, when compared with the surrounding parenchyma, with poorly defined margins. Clinical history plays an important role in helping to differentiate focal orchitis from an actual mass. The presence of

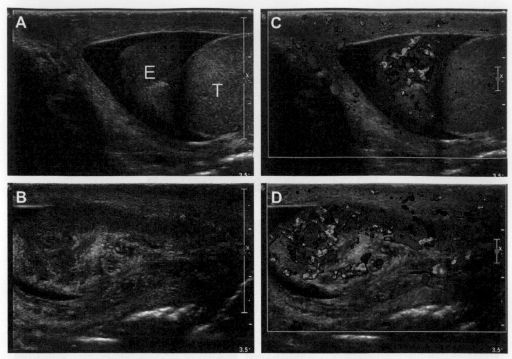

Fig. 13. Gray-scale (*A, B*) and color Doppler (*C, D*) ultrasonographic images obtained in a patient with acute epididymitis, demonstrate an enlarged heterogeneous epididymis (E) with increased vascularity and a small amount of surrounding fluid. The testicle (T) is normal in echogenicity and vascularity.

pain, fever, and coexistent infection of the epididymis all favor focal orchitis. Besides primary testicular tumors, leukemia and lymphoma can have similar appearances, and therefore, follow-up to complete resolution should be performed with focal abnormalities to rule out malignancy.[17] Orchitis is often associated with a reactive hydrocele as well as scrotal wall thickening and

hyperemia. Complications of orchitis include intratesticular abscess formation (**Fig. 16**), testicular infarction, pyocele, and ultimately, if left untreated, infertility.

It is important to remember to always compare the affected epididymis or testis to the normal side because the findings may be subtle and may only be appreciated qualitatively.

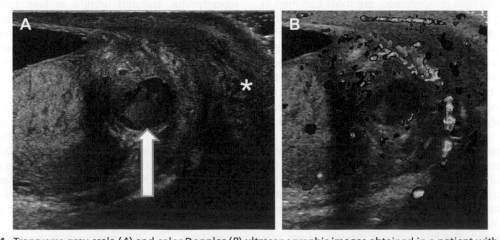

Fig. 14. Transverse gray-scale (*A*) and color Doppler (*B*) ultrasonographic images obtained in a patient with acute scrotal pain, swelling, and fever demonstrate an enlarged and heterogeneous epididymal tail with increased vascularity and a focal abscess (*arrow, A*). Also note extensive scrotal wall thickening (*asterisk, A*) and increased vascularity.

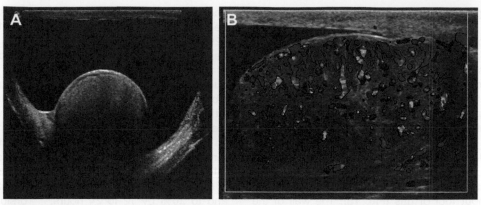

Fig. 15. Gray-scale (*A*) and color Doppler (*B*) ultrasonographic images obtained in a patient with acute orchitis demonstrate a heterogeneous testis with increased vascularity and a large complex hydrocele.

Scrotal wall infections

Fournier gangrene is a rapidly progressive, infectious necrotizing fasciitis of the perineal, perianal, and genital regions with a mortality rate of 15% to 50% and is considered a urological emergency.[19] Inflammation and edema from infection result in an impaired local blood supply, leading to vascular thrombosis. The infection spreads rapidly through the subcutaneous soft tissues and fascial planes, ultimately leading to gangrene. Early diagnosis is important because immediate surgical debridement and aggressive antibiotic treatment are necessary. Skin infections can lead to abscess formation in the perineal or perianal regions, whereas urological sources of infection include chronic urinary tract infections, uretheral strictures, epididymitis, and neurogenic bladder.[20]

Additional sources of infection can arise from colon perforation, diverticulitis, and even rectal cancer.[21] Fournier gangrene is caused by a polymicrobial infection with the most common bacteria including *E coli*, *Bacteroides*, and streptococcal and staphylococcus species. Fournier gangrene is most commonly seen in middle-aged men but can also occur in women and children. There are several conditions that predispose the patient to the development of Fournier gangrene, such as diabetes, immunosuppression, alcohol abuse and cirrhosis, and morbid obesity. Although the diagnosis is made clinically, radiological imaging can help confirm and evaluate the extent of disease. Imaging of Fournier gangrene can be performed with radiographs, CT, and/or ultrasonography. The most important finding on all 3

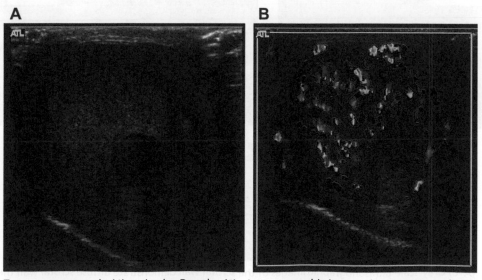

Fig. 16. Transverse gray-scale (*A*) and color Doppler (*B*) ultrasonographic images demonstrate an intratesticular abscess with a fluid-fluid level, increased vascularity, and small amount of surrounding fluid.

imaging modalities is the presence of subcutaneous gas. On ultrasonography, subcutaneous gas appears as discrete hyperechoic foci with "dirty" posterior shadowing (**Fig. 17**).[22] In addition to the subcutaneous foci of gas, scrotal wall thickening can be seen on gray-scale imaging, with hyperemia on color imaging. Ultrasonography is probably the most sensitive modality for small amounts of gas, whereas CT is best to evaluate the full extent of the disease, particularly any intraperitoneal spread.

A scrotal wall abscess appears as a well-circumscribed, complex hypoechoic region with or without foci of gas (**Fig. 18**). The wall of the abscess has an echogenic rim with variable thickness. As with other infections of the scrotum, scrotal wall thickening and hyperemia are also often present. Scrotal wall abscesses can be directly caused by infection of hair follicles or sweat glands or abrasions of the skin.[23] They can also be caused by underlying infections of the epididymis or testis, with spread to the scrotal wall.

Scrotal wall cellulitis appears as diffuse scrotal wall thickening with increased vascularity in the underlying soft tissues but without a focal fluid collection. The subcutaneous tissues appear hypoechoic, secondary to edema.

Testicular Torsion

Testicular torsion is defined as a twist of the spermatic cord or of the testis itself on its attachments.

The extent of testicular ischemia depends on the degree of torsion, which ranges from 180° to 720° or greater.[17] The testicular salvage rate depends on the degree of torsion and the duration of ischemia.[17] The first hemodynamic consequence of testicular torsion is venous obstruction. Obstruction of arterial inflow follows because the intratesticular pressure increases, and eventually, testicular ischemia occurs. Infarction can occur as soon as 4 hours after the appearance of symptoms. Reports show that a nearly 100% salvage rate exists within the first 6 hours after the onset of symptoms; diminishing to 70% at 6 to 12 hours and to 20% by 12 to 24 hours.[24] Torsion most commonly occurs as a result of an anatomic anomaly known as the bell-clapper deformity. In this setting, the tunica vaginalis completely encircles the epididymis, the distal spermatic cord, and the testis. This deformity allows the testis to freely suspend in the scrotum and more easily twist and rotate within the tunica vaginalis, like a clapper in a bell.[17]

The radiologist should first examine the patient to look for clues to the presence of torsion visually, such as an elevated position or horizontal alignment of the affected testicle. Gray-scale images are nonspecific for testicular torsion and may be normal if the torsion has just occurred.[17] Gray-scale abnormalities include decreased testicular echogenicity, testicular enlargement, scrotal wall thickening, and a reactive hydrocele (**Fig. 19**). In some cases, the actual twisting of the spermatic

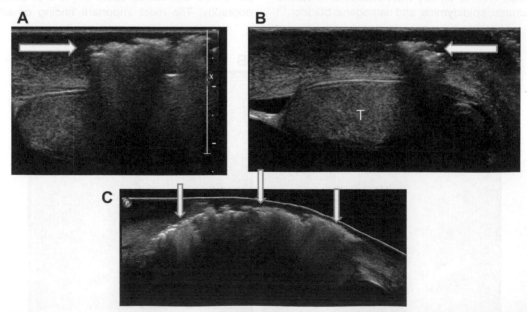

Fig. 17. (A–C) Gray-scale ultrasonographic images of the scrotal wall demonstrate diffuse scrotal wall thickening and extensive subcutaneous air (*arrows*) in this patient with surgically proven Fournier gangrene. The testis (T) is normal.

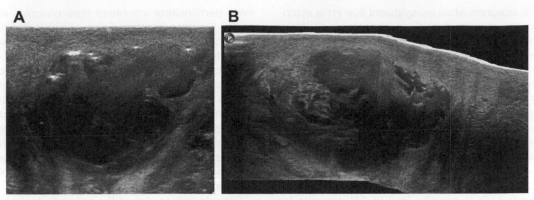

Fig. 18. Longitudinal (*A*) and panoramic gray-scale (*B*) ultrasonographic images demonstrate a large complex fluid collection with foci of gas in the subcutaneous soft tissues representing a scrotal wall abscess.

cord can be appreciated sonographically. In a study by Baud and colleagues,[25] a spiral twisting of the spermatic cord at the external inguinal ring was seen in 14 of 23 cases of torsion. In the setting of acute torsion, with normal echogenicity, the testis is likely to be viable regardless of the duration of symptoms. If there is acute torsion with hemorrhagic infarction, the testis appears hyperechoic and heterogeneous. Chronic infarction results in an atrophic hypoechoic testis, often

with calcification. Because gray-scale ultrasonographic findings can be normal in the early phase of torsion, the Doppler component of the examination is essential.

The absence of testicular flow at color and power Doppler ultrasonography is considered diagnostic of ischemia. Asymmetrically decreased vascularity and an increased resistive index on the affected side are also signs of testicular torsion. Doppler examination is 86% sensitive, 100% specific, and

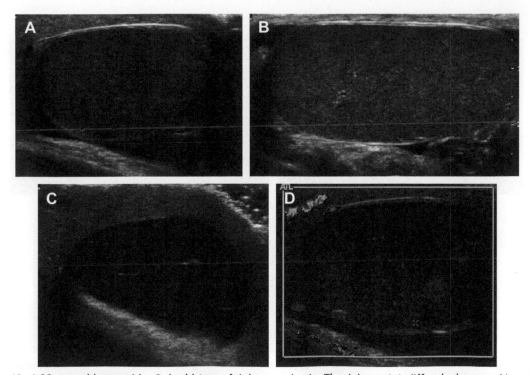

Fig. 19. A 28-year-old man with a 3-day history of right scrotal pain. The right testis is diffusely decreased in echogenicity (*A*) when compared with the normal left testis (*B*). (*C*) A reactive right-sided hydrocele with a thin internal septation. (*D*) No blood flow within the right testis on color Doppler imaging, consistent with testicular torsion. At the time of surgery, the testis was found to be infarcted.

97% accurate when using absent flow in the symptomatic side as the diagnostic criteria.[26] When evaluating for testicular torsion, it is essential that the ultrasonographic technique be optimized for detection of slow flow, including use of the smallest appropriate color sampling box with adjustments for the lowest pulse repetition frequency and the lowest possible threshold setting.[27] Power Doppler is especially valuable in scrotal sonography because of its increased sensitivity to low-flow states and its independence from the Doppler angle correction.[28] Yagil and colleagues[29] demonstrated that Doppler ultrasonography was 94% sensitive, 96% specific, and 95.5% accurate for the diagnosis of testicular torsion with a positive predictive value (PPV) of 89.4% and a negative predictive value (NPV) of 98%.

However, the presence of flow does not exclude torsion. Testicular torsion is not an all-or-none phenomenon. Partial torsion, transient torsion, and torsion-detorsion are well known entities. Asymmetry in resistive indices with decreased diastolic flow or diastolic flow reversal may be seen in partial torsion; however, there are no studies to validate the role of spectral Doppler ultrasonography in partial torsion.[28] If the testis is scanned shortly after detorsion, the affected testis may even demonstrate increased flow on color and power Doppler imaging. False-negative findings can occur in the setting of intermittent or low-grade torsion or with spontaneous detorsion.

Anecdotally, the radiologist can have not only a diagnostic but also a therapeutic effect in the setting of acute testicular torsion. In the authors' opinion, if there is no flow within the testis and if the gray-scale findings remain normal, the radiologist can attempt to manually detorse the affected testicle. Immediately after manual detorsion, blood flow should be reestablished to the testis with relative peripheral hyperemia (Fig. 20).

Patients with torsion of the appendix testis and appendix epididymis also present with acute scrotal pain. The classic finding at physical examination is a small firm palpable nodule on the superior aspect of the testis with bluish discoloration of the overlying skin, called the "blue dot" sign.[17] Although torsion of an appendage is a clinical diagnosis, ultrasonography usually reveals a hyperechoic mass with a central hypoechoic area adjacent to the testis or epididymis. Reactive hydroceles and skin thickening are common in these cases. Increased peripheral flow may be seen around the twisted testicular appendage at color Doppler ultrasonography.[30]

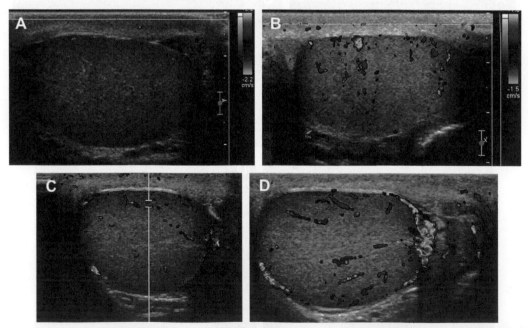

Fig. 20. Torsion-detorsion. Longitudinal color Doppler images of the right (A) and left (B) testes, in a patient with acute right scrotal pain, demonstrate no blood flow in the right testis, with normal flow in the left testis, consistent with acute right testicular torsion. The right testis remains normal in echogenicity. Color Doppler images of the right testis, immediately after manual detorsion (C, D) demonstrate reconstitution of blood flow within the testis and peripheral hyperemia.

Trauma

Trauma is the third most common cause of acute scrotal pain, and ultrasonography plays an important role in assessing the severity of injury and triaging patients for surgical versus nonsurgical management.[31] Significant testicular injuries can occur without external signs, and a negative ultrasonographic result should not preclude surgery in cases in which there is a high risk or a high degree of suspicion.[31] The 3 causes of scrotal injury are blunt trauma, penetrating trauma, and iatrogenic injuries. Sporting activities account for more than half of all cases of testicular injury, and motor vehicle accidents are responsible for another 9% to 17% of testicular injuries.[31] Penetrating injuries are most commonly secondary to gunshot wounds, stab wounds, or bites.

Ultrasonography is extremely sensitive for disruption of the testis. Buckley and McAnintch[32] reported a sensitivity of 100% and a specificity of 93.5% for the diagnosis of testicular rupture. The 4 important sonographic findings of testicular rupture include discontinuity of the tunica albuginea, abnormal contour of the testis, heterogeneous echotexture of the testis, and absence of vascularity in the testis.[31] The most definitive finding is direct demonstration of a discontinuity in the tunica albuginea in a patient with a history of scrotal trauma.[31] The other 3 findings, if present, provide additional support to the diagnosis of testicular rupture. The abnormal contour of the testis is caused by the extrusion of testicular parenchyma,

after disruption of the tunica albuginea (**Fig. 21**).[33] The heterogeneous echotexture results from edema and hemorrhage. Color Doppler imaging is important to evaluate for viability.

Intratesticular hematomas occurring in the setting of blunt trauma have a variable appearance, based on chronicity. Acute intratesticular hematomas may be difficult to visualize because they are often isoechoic to the testis. Therefore, it is recommended that suspected acute hematomas be reimaged in 12 to 24 hours after the initial ultrasonography in order to evaluate for changes.[33] Subacute hematomas are more heterogeneous (**Fig. 22**), and chronic intratesticular hematomas are hypoechoic and may contain septations, debris, or fluid-fluid levels representing the various stages of blood products. The history of trauma is crucial because the appearance may overlap with an abscess. Hematomas can also vary in size and number. A testicular contusion appears as a focal area of decreased echogenicity, when compared with the surrounding parenchyma, with less-well defined borders than a hematoma or abscess. Color and pulsed Doppler imaging reveals decreased flow in the area of contusion.

A hematocele is a collection of blood within the tunica vaginalis and is the most common finding in the scrotum after a blunt trauma. Acute hematoceles are typically hyperechoic or isoechoic to the testicular parenchyma. Chronic hematoceles are hypoechoic, may contain internal septations or fluid-fluid levels, and may even calcify. If

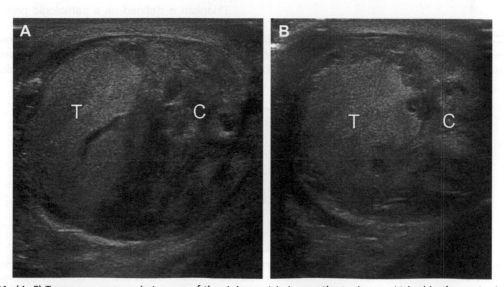

Fig. 21. (*A, B*) Transverse gray-scale images of the right testicle in a patient who was kicked in the groin demonstrate diffuse irregularity of the contour of the testis (T) and a large heterogeneous collection (C) compressing the testis. Surgery revealed disruption of the tunica albuginea, extrusion of testicular parenchyma, and hematoma.

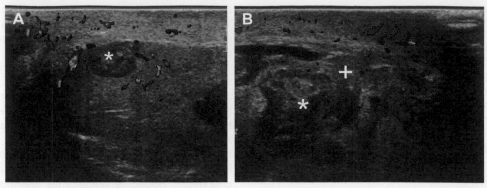

Fig. 22. (A, B) A 35-year-old man with a history of scrotal trauma 2 days prior. Longitudinal color Doppler ultrasonographic images demonstrate focal intratesticular hematomas (*asterisk*) and extrusion of testicular parenchyma through a disruption in the tunica albuginea (*plus, B*).

a hematocele becomes large enough, it can cause mass effect on the testis and reduce blood flow (**Fig. 23**), in which case surgical evacuation is necessary to relieve the pressure and prevent testicular ischemia. In fact, the presence of a large hematocele is an indication for surgery because of the limited capability of ultrasonography to visualize a rupture of the tunica albuginea in the presence of surrounding complex fluid.[31]

A fracture of the testis can appear as a hypoechoic avascular line through the testis. Visualization of a fracture line is rare and has been reported in only 17% of cases.[17]

Additional findings seen in penetrating injuries, but not in blunt trauma, include foci of air within the scrotum and testis, an intratesticular missile track, and the presence of foreign bodies (**Fig. 24**).[32]

Penile Pain

Differential considerations for men who present with acute penile pain include priapism, trauma, infection/inflammation, and dorsal vein thrombosis. Patients who have had trauma to the penis present with severe pain, swelling, and deformity of the penile shaft. The trauma most often occurs during sexual intercourse but can also occur from falling on an erect penis. Multiple imaging modalities are used in the setting of pelvic trauma to evaluate for injuries to the urinary tract, including CT, CT cystography, and retrograde urethrography. However, in isolated injuries to the penis, ultrasonography provides a quick evaluation for disruption of the tunica albuginea, hematoma, and penile vascular injuries. The most important finding in determining the need for surgery is the integrity of the tunica albuginea (**Fig. 25**).[34] If unrepaired, penile fractures can lead to a permanent deformity and erectile dysfunction.

Priapism is defined as a pathologic prolonged penile erection that is unrelated to sexual arousal and is separated into 2 types: high flow (nonischemic) and low flow (ischemic). The most commonly encountered type of priapism is the ischemic type

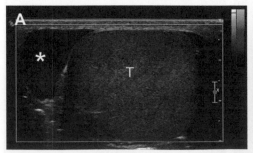
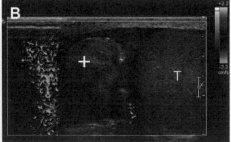

Fig. 23. Power (A) and color (B) Doppler ultrasonographic images of the right testis in a patient who sustained significant trauma to the scrotum, demonstrate no detectable blood flow within the testis (T) that remains normal in echogenicity. A hematocele (*asterisk, A*) and large hematoma (*plus, B*) are partially visualized. At the time of surgery, the testicle was initially blue. After clearing out the hematoma and hematocele, there was good flow and viability of the right testis.

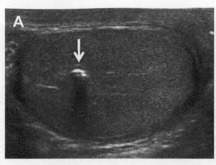
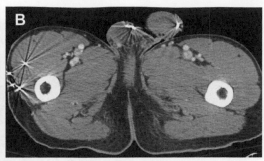

Fig. 24. Longitudinal gray-scale ultrasonographic image (*A*) demonstrates a linear brightly echogenic focus within the testis with posterior shadowing (*arrow*). CT (*B*) demonstrates multiple metallic foreign bodies throughout the soft tissues in this patient who was shot with birdshot.

in which men present with a prolonged, painful erection. Low-flow priapism and the associated severe decrease in venous drainage from the corpora cavernosa is a potential medical emergency because it can lead to irreversible ischemic changes.[35] The most common cause of low-flow priapism is an intracavernosal injection of vasoactive agents, such as papaverine or prostaglandin. Risk factors for developing priapism include hemoglobinopathies such as sickle cell disease, cocaine use, and certain antipsychotic medications, such as trazodone, thioridazine, and chlorpromazine. Patients with metastatic disease to the penis or direct spread from advanced pelvic cancers can develop malignant priapism. High-flow priapism is less common, and patients typically present with a painless erection, most commonly secondary to perineal or penile trauma and resultant arteriosinusoidal malformation.

Ultrasonography plays an important role as the first imaging modality to differentiate between the 2 types of priapism and to evaluate for the extent of disease. Hakim and colleagues[36] showed that penile Doppler sonography has a sensitivity of 100%, a specificity of 73%, a PPV of 81%, and an NPV of 100%. Ultrasonography is a noninvasive way to differentiate between ischemic and nonischemic priapism, instead of blood gas sampling that requires needle aspiration.[34] Color and pulsed Doppler imaging are used to evaluate for patency of the cavernosal arteries as well as detailed evaluation of the blood flow including waveforms and peak systolic and end-diastolic velocities. In general, patients with ischemic priapism have minimal or absent blood flow in the cavernosal arteries (**Fig. 26**), whereas patients with nonischemic priapism typically have increased arterial blood flow and a history of perineal/penile trauma causing an arteriosinusoidal fistula. On gray-scale imaging, tissue edema causes an increase in echogenicity throughout the corpora cavernosa, whereas prolonged priapism causes ischemic changes and fibrosis, which appears as a coarsening in the echotexture.[34]

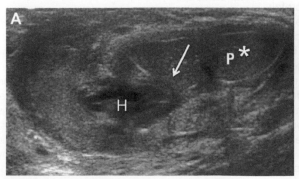
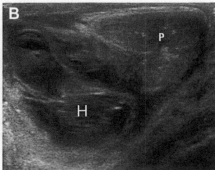

Fig. 25. (*A*, *B*) Transverse gray-scale ultrasonographic images of the penis (P) in a patient with acute penile trauma demonstrate disruption of the tunica albuginea surrounding the right corpora cavernosum (*arrow*, *A*) and a large soft tissue hematoma (H). The tunica albuginea surrounding the left corpora cavernosum (*asterisk*, *A*) is intact.

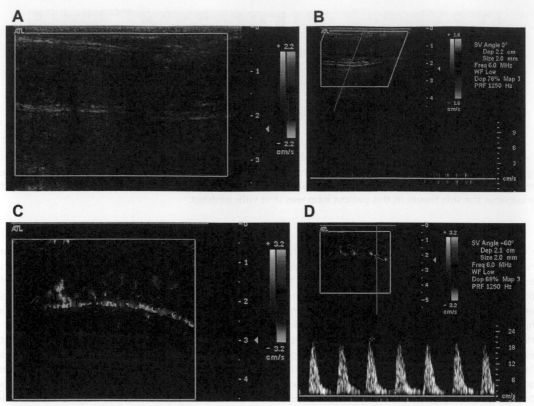

Fig. 26. Color (*A*) and pulsed Doppler (*B*) ultrasonographic images of the left cavernosal artery demonstrate no blood flow within the vessel in a patient with a prolonged, painful erection. No flow was present in the right cavernosal artery as well. Four days after placement of a penile shunt, color (*C*) and pulsed Doppler (*D*) ultrasonographic images demonstrate flow in the left cavernosal artery with a normal arterial waveform. Similar findings were also present in the right cavernosal artery.

SUMMARY

Ultrasonography is the primary imaging modality for the evaluation of acute scrotal pain and plays a critical role in differentiating between causes that require urgent surgical intervention, such as testicular torsion, and causes that can be treated medically. The ability to image the scrotal contents in real time with color and spectral Doppler, the ready availability, and the lack of ionizing radiation, make ultrasonography ideal for evaluating the male genitalia in the emergency setting. Although CT is the most commonly used imaging modality for the kidneys and bladder in the emergency setting, considerations of contrast and radiation dose warrant the use of ultrasonography as a primary imaging modality in certain situations (ie, children, pregnant women, and patients who have had multiple prior CTs for repeated episodes of renal colic). Detailed clinical information can guide the sonographer to search for specific diagnoses, using color and spectral Doppler. Equipped with the knowledge of the

sonographic features and using meticulous technique, a broad spectrum of diseases affecting the genitourinary tract can be confidently diagnosed with ultrasonography.

REFERENCES

1. Kambadakone AR, Eisner BH, Onofrio AC, et al. New and evolving concepts in the imaging and management of urolithiasis: urologists' perspective. Radiographics 2010;30:603–23.
2. Sheafor DH, Hertzberg BS, Freed KS, et al. Nonenhanced helical CT and US in the emergency evaluation of patients with renal colic: prospective comparison. Radiology 2000;217:792–7.
3. Park SJ, Yi BH, Lee HK, et al. Evaluation of patients with suspected ureteral calculi using sonography as an initial diagnostic tool: how can we improve diagnostic accuracy? J Ultrasound Med 2008;27:1441–50.
4. Patlas M, Farkas A, Fisher D, et al. Ultrasound vs CT for the detection of ureteric stones in patients with renal colic. Br J Radiol 2001;74:901–4.

5. Ripolles T, Agramunt M, Errando J, et al. Suspected ureteral colic: plain film and sonography vs unenhanced helical CT. A prospective study in 66 patients. Eur Radiol 2004;14:129–36.

6. Mitterberger M, Pinggera GM, Maier E, et al. Value of 3-dimensional transrectal/transvaginal sonography in diagnosis of distal ureteral calculi. J Ultrasound Med 2007;26:19–27.

7. Durr-E-Sabih, Khan AN, Craig M, et al. Sonographic mimics of renal calculi. J Ultrasound Med 2004;23: 1361–7.

8. Lee JY, Kim SH, Cho JY, et al. Color and power Doppler twinkling artifacts from urinary stones: clinical observations and phantom studies. AJR Am J Roentgenol 2001;176:1441–5.

9. Burge HJ, Middleton WD, McClennan BL, et al. Ureteral jets in healthy subjects and in patients with unilateral ureteral calculi: comparison with color Doppler US. Radiology 1991;180:437–42.

10. Tublin ME, Bude RO, Platt JF. The resistive index in renal Doppler sonography: where do we stand? AJR Am J Roentgenol 2003;180:885–92.

11. Farmer KD, Gellett LR. The sonographic appearance of acute focal pyelonephritis: 8 years' experience. Clin Radiol 2002;57:483–7.

12. Cavorsi K, Prabhakar P, Kirby C. Acute pyelonephritis. Ultrasound Q 2010;26:103–5.

13. Korner M, Krotz MM, Degenhart C, et al. Current role of emergency US in patients with major trauma. Radiographics 2008;28:225–44.

14. Kim KW, Kim M, Kim H, et al. Value of "patent track" sign on Doppler sonography after percutaneous liver biopsy in detection of postbiopsy bleeding: a prospective study in 352 patients. AJR Am J Roentgenol 2007;189:109–16.

15. Lockhart ME, Wells CG, Morgan DE, et al. Reversed diastolic flow in the renal transplant: perioperative implications versus transplants older than 1 month. AJR Am J Roentgenol 2008;190:650–5.

16. Correas J, Claudon M, Tranquart F, et al. The kidney: imaging with microbubble contrast agents. Ultrasound Q 2006;22:53–66.

17. Dogra VS, Gottlieb RH, Oka M, et al. Sonography of the scrotum. Radiology 2003;227:18–36.

18. Horstman WG, Middleton WD, Melson GL. Scrotal inflammatory disease: color Doppler ultrasound findings. Radiology 1991;179:55–9.

19. Levenson RB, Singh AK, Novelline RA. Fournier gangrene: role of imaging. Radiographics 2008;28: 519–28.

20. Amdendola MA, Casillas J, Joseph R, et al. Fournier's gangrene: CT findings. Abdom Imaging 1994;19:471–4.

21. Ash L, Hale J. CT findings in perforated rectal carcinoma presenting as Fournier's gangrene in the emergency department. Emerg Radiol 2005;11: 295–7.

22. Rajan DK, Scharer KA. Radiology of Fournier's gangrene. AJR Am J Roentgenol 1998;170:163–8.

23. Berman JM, Beidle TR, Kunberger LE, et al. Sonographic evaluation of acute intrascrotal pathology. AJR Am J Roentgenol 1996;166:857–61.

24. Patriquin HB, Yazbeck S, Trinh B, et al. Testicular torsion in infants and children: diagnosis with Doppler sonography. Radiology 1993;188:781–5.

25. Baud C, Veyrae C, Couture A, et al. Spiral twist of the spermatic cord: a reliable sign of testicular torsion. Pediatr Radiol 1998;28:950–4.

26. Burks DD, Markey BJ, Burkhard TK, et al. Suspected testicular torsion and ischemia: evaluation with color Doppler sonography. Radiology 1990;175:815–21.

27. Wilbert DM, Schaerfe CW, Stern WD, et al. Evaluation of the acute scrotum by color-coded Doppler ultrasonography. J Urol 1993;149:1475–7.

28. Dogra VS, Bhatt S, Rubens D. Sonographic evaluation of testicular torsion. Ultrasound Clin 2006;1: 55–66.

29. Yagil Y, Naroditsky I, Milhem J, et al. Role of Doppler ultrasonography in the triage of acute scrotum in the emergency department. J Ultrasound Med 2010;29: 11–21.

30. Cohen HL, Shapiro MA, Haller JO, et al. Torsion of the testicular appendage: sonographic diagnosis. J Ultrasound Med 1992;11:81–3.

31. Bhatt S, Dogra VS. Role of US in testicular and scrotal trauma. Radiographics 2008;28:1617–29.

32. Buckley JC, McAnintch JW. Use of ultrasonography for the diagnosis of testicular injuries in blunt scrotal trauma. J Urol 2006;175:175–8.

33. Bhatt S, Ghazale H, Dogra VS. Sonographic evaluation of scrotal and penile trauma. Ultrasound Clin 2007;2:45–56.

34. Bertolotto M, Pavlica P, Serafini G, et al. Painful penile induration: imaging findings and management. Radiographics 2009;29:477–93.

35. Sadeghi-Nejad H, Dogra V, Seftel AD, et al. Priapism. Radiol Clin North Am 2004;42:427–43.

36. Hakim LS, Kulaksizoglu H, Mulligan R, et al. Evolving concepts in the diagnosis and treatment of arterial high flow priapism. J Urol 1996;155:541.

Common Applications of Musculoskeletal Ultrasound in the Emergency Department

Ghaneh Fananapazir, MD[a],*, Sandra J. Allison, MD[b]

KEYWORDS
• Ultrasound • Musculoskeletal • Emergency
• Tendon • Ligament • Muscle

Owing to its portability and real-time capability, ultrasound is extremely well suited for evaluating patients who present to the emergency department. With ultrasound, one can address and often answer a focused clinical question in a timely manner. This is invaluable in unstable trauma settings where patients cannot be transported from their rooms.

The superficial location of tendons, ligaments, muscles, nerves, and superficial soft tissues of the extremities lends itself to sonographic imaging. Other musculoskeletal applications of ultrasound in the emergency department include evaluating for fluid collections, detecting soft tissue foreign bodies, particularly radiolucent ones, and, in certain instances, diagnosing bony fractures.

TECHNIQUE

For scanning the extremity, a high-frequency (9–17 MHz) linear array transducer is the most appropriate choice. Proper positioning of the patient is essential to obtaining high-quality images. The goal is to keep the patient comfortable yet allow a dynamic examination to be performed. Comparison with the unaffected contralateral extremity can be made. Color and power Doppler sonography can be used to assess the degree of vascularity and characterize inflammation. The dynamic portion of the examination can be recorded with cine so that transient conditions related to specific positions or movements can be reviewed after the examination. Widescreen, panoramic, and split-screen functions can expand the field of view. In the setting of unstable trauma or in patients experiencing significant pain, the examination can be tailored to specifically address the clinical question. In less emergent situations, a more comprehensive examination can be performed. The most important part of the examination, however, is interaction with the patient. The precise location and character of symptoms can be discussed with the patient. The probe can then be placed directly over that location to palpate for tenderness and correlate with or assist in interpretation of the findings.

The extremity structures that can be evaluated with ultrasound and common pathology that may be encountered in the setting of the emergency department are discussed in the following sections.

This work was not supported by grants.
The authors have nothing to disclose.
[a] Department of Radiology, Georgetown University Hospital, 3800 Reservoir Road, NW, Washington, DC 20007-2113, USA
[b] Division of Ultrasound, Department of Radiology, Georgetown University Hospital, 3800 Reservoir Road, NW, Washington, DC 20007-2113, USA
* Corresponding author.
E-mail address: gxf105@gunet.georgetown.edu

Ultrasound Clin 6 (2011) 215–226
doi:10.1016/j.cult.2011.03.001

TENDONS

A tendon is a band of connective tissue that connects a muscle with its bony attachment. It is composed of type I collagen fibrils oriented in parallel planes in the longitudinal direction. The superficiality of most tendons allows for excellent visualization by ultrasound. Sonographically, the parallel fibrillar lines appear echogenic in the longitudinal direction and as dotlike echogenic structures in the transverse plane. The tendon is surrounded by a paratenon or by a synovial sheath. The surrounding sheaths contain a small amount of fluid that usually appears anechoic.[1] Many tendons also have an adjacent bursa.

Tendons, on the longitudinal views, appear as echogenic parallel lines. An artifact can be produced if the transducer is slightly angulated in which a portion of the tendon will appear hypoechoic, mimicking tendon pathology. This is referred to as anisotropy. If the hypoechoic-appearing tendon is attributable to anisotropy, minor changes in angulation will eventually show the continuity of the echogenic tendon. However, if it reflects true pathology, normal echogenicity will not be demonstrated regardless of the angulation.[2]

Tendon Tears/Rupture/Avulsion

A tear involving a normal tendon is rare and usually occurs only in the setting of severe trauma. Most tendon ruptures occur in tendons with underlying tendinopathy that weakens the tendon, resulting in tears from even minor tendon strains.[2] Tendinopathy can predispose to partial tendon tears, which can lead to full-thickness tears, with fluid, hemorrhage, or intervening herniated tissue in tendon defect.[3] Both tendinosis and partial-thickness tears are usually treated conservatively, whereas full-thickness tears may benefit from surgical management.

Complete tendon tears represent a complete disruption in all the parallel fibrillar lines, with the proximal tendon end retracted, appearing blunted or frayed. On transverse views, the blunted end appears rounded and masslike. Posterior shadowing at the proximal tendon can be observed and does not necessarily represent avulsed bone, but rather be attributable to refraction. Decreased echogenicity in the tendon at the retracted end or along any portion of the tendon may be related to buckling or change in alignment of the fibers resulting in anisotropy. There can be an adjacent fluid collection, which represents fluid or a hematoma, usually at the musculotendinous junction. A tendon sheath effusion may also be present. Avulsed bony fragments can occur at tendinous insertions and appear as echogenic structures attached to the tendon. Locating the ends of a full-thickness tear can be challenging with the intervening hemorrhage or approximation of torn tendon ends. In this setting, color or power Doppler can be useful.[4] Partial-thickness tears, on the other hand, can be seen as disruption of the internal fibrillar architecture, with at least some maintenance of the fibrillar lines. There is no retraction in partial tears. Hemorrhage or fluid can also be seen filling the intervening portion.

Overuse of a tendon can lead to degenerative changes, which can predispose to partial and full-length tears. In this setting, the term tendinosis is preferred to tendonitis, as there are no acute inflammatory cells within the affected tendon.[5] Symptoms may mimic those of tendon tears. Sonographic changes include diffuse thickening and relative decreased echogenicity of the involved tendon and may demonstrate increased blood flow on power Doppler imaging, which is a result of neovascularization rather than an inflammatory recruitment of vascular flow. If the synovium is involved, as it often is, it is termed tenosynovitis. Overuse of a tendon can lead to edema, fluid, or synovitis in the synovial sheath, paratenon, or adjacent bursae.[2] Sonographic features include fluid distension of the synovial tendon sheath, either in a diffuse or eccentric manner, and thickening of the sheath itself.

Achilles Tendon Rupture

The Achilles tendon represents the most common site of tendon rupture.[3] The most typical location for injury is 4 to 6 cm proximal to the calcaneus. Both biomechanical and vascular factors have been postulated to account for the predisposition for this location.[2] Early changes of tendinosis in the Achilles tendon include increased fluid in the paratenon and decreased echogenicity of the tendon. Partial tears can be visualized as partial-thickness loss of normal fibrillation. Ultrasound images can be obtained with the patient in dorsiflexion and plantarflexion, improving visualization of partial-thickness tears. Intervening hemorrhage and fluid can be seen in complete tendon tears (**Fig. 1**). Loss of plantarflexion can imply a complete Achilles tendon rupture. However, complete rupture can also be seen in a patient who is able to plantarflex if the plantaris tendon is intact.[2]

Patellar Tendon Rupture

The patellar tendon attaches from the lower pole of the patella to the tibial tuberosity. A common precursor to patellar tendon rupture is a condition called "jumper's knee," usually seen in athletes

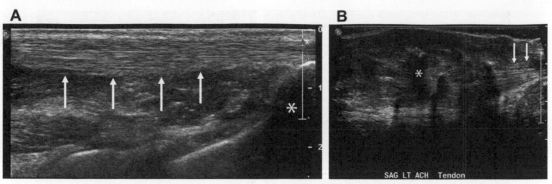

Fig. 1. Achilles tendon re-rupture. (*A*) Long axis view of the heel (in a different patient) showing a normal Achilles tendon (*arrows*) inserting on the calcaneus (*asterisk*). Note the fine parallel echogenic lines that make up the tendon. (*B*) Scan of a patient who presented to the emergency department after experiencing tearing pain in the area of prior Achilles repair. Most of the tendon is disrupted and heterogeneous material representing hematoma is filling the area of tear (*asterisk*). A small portion of intact tendon is seen distally (*arrows*).

who engage in activities or exercises that require rapid and repetitive contraction of the quadriceps muscles. The injury involves microtears in the patellar tendon, near the inferior patellar insertion. Patients with jumper's knee usually initially complain of pain at the inferior patellar insertion immediately after exercise, which can progress to chronic nonexercise-induced pain, and finally to frank rupture. Sonographically, jumper's knee can appear as a central hypoechogenic region in the proximal posterior portion of the patellar tendon.[6] If more chronic in nature, dystrophic calcifications can occur at the region of the patellar insertion. Usually, tears of the patellar tendon are partial, presenting sonographically as a hypoechogenic focus within the patellar tendon. Rarely, a full tendon rupture of the patellar tendon will occur, usually in the setting of an acute traumatic injury on a background of more chronic injury.

Biceps Tendon

The long head of the biceps brachii tendon is located between the greater and lesser tuberosities of the proximal humerus in a region called the bicipital groove. It enters the glenohumeral joint through a region called the rotator interval, which is a space between the supraspinatus and subscapularis tendons. The long head of the biceps brachii tendon is stabilized by the bicipital sulcus with a roofing composed of, from superior to inferior, the coracohumeral ligament, superior glenohumeral ligament, transverse humeral ligament, and the pectoralis major muscle.[7]

As with other tendons, the ultrasound appearance of tendinosis is hypoechoic enlargement of the tendon without disruption of the tendon fibers. Partial tears demonstrate anechoic clefts within the tendon. Full-thickness tendon tears lead to a more distal retraction of the long head of the biceps tendon, leading to an empty bicipital groove, which may be filled with fluid or hemorrhage. Hyperechoic hemorrhage within the bicipital groove should not be confused with tendon fibers. The tendon should be evaluated more distally, which will appear retracted into a stump.[8] Lack of visualization of the long head of the biceps tendon may indicate a complete disruption of the tendon, but may also indicate a subluxed or dislocated tendon. Forcible contraction of the biceps or external rotation of the shoulder can lead to medial displacement of the biceps tendon.[7] This usually occurs with a tear of the coracohumeral ligament or the subscapularis tendon. Maneuvers can be of assistance, as some subluxations or dislocations can be observed only with the shoulder in external rotation.[7]

Plantaris Tendon Tear

A form of "tennis leg" is injury to the plantaris tendon. The plantaris muscle is often considered vestigial, weakly plantarflexing the foot. It is congenitally absent in approximately 10% of the population. The plantaris muscle has its proximal attachment at the inferior lateral supracondylar ridge of the femur, just superior to the attachment of the lateral head of the gastrocnemius. The tendon travels inferomedially, inserting onto the calcaneus. The tendon can be visualized sonographically between the gastrocnemius and soleus muscles (**Fig. 2**A). Tears usually occur at the level of the mid-calf. Disruption of the plantaris tendon can demonstrate a tubular fluid collection between the gastrocnemius and soleus muscles (see **Fig.** 2B). Gastrocnemius tears can also produce fluid in this region, and a plantaris tear

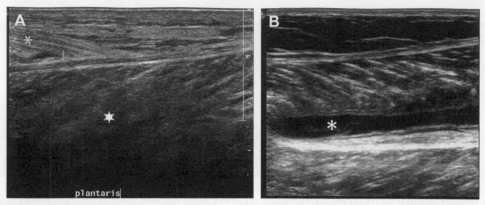

Fig. 2. Plantaris tendon rupture. (*A*) Long axis view of a normal plantaris tendon (*arrow*) located between the gastrocnemius (*asterisk*) and soleus (*star*) muscles. (*B*) Tubular fluid collection (*asterisk*) located between the gastrocnemius and soleus muscles in a patient who experienced an acute plantaris rupture. The plantaris tendon was not seen.

and gastrocnemius tear can often coexist.[4] Both conditions present with calf pain and in the emergency department may lead to a search for lower extremity deep venous thrombosis. Knowledge of these conditions may clue the sonographer into assessing these areas in the calf in patients presenting with classic history and symptoms.

Finger Tendon Laceration

Injuries to the flexor tendons of the hand are common and often will present as an emergency because of the important role the hands play in labor and everyday activities. In the acute setting, tendon laceration can be difficult to diagnose by physical examination alone since pain can limit the range of motion. Digital swelling and the

presence of a hematoma may cause finger stiffness, further limiting range of motion.

Although ultrasound may not be reliable at distinguishing partial-thickness tears from anisotropy, ultrasound is useful at identifying full-thickness tears of the extensor and flexor tendons of the fingers (**Fig. 3**).

LIGAMENTS

Ligaments are also composed of type I collagen, connecting bone with bone. Similar to tendons, ligaments appear as bright parallel lines on longitudinal views and as dotlike echogenic structures on the transverse images. However, ligaments are often more difficult to image at 90 degrees

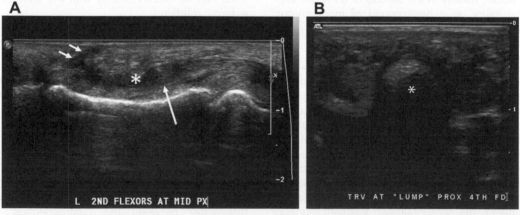

Fig. 3. Flexor digitorum profunda tendon (FDP) laceration. (*A*) Longitudinal scan of the palmar surface of the left second digit in a patient who experienced a laceration with a box cutter and subsequent loss of function demonstrates an empty tendon sheath (*asterisk*). The tendon is retracted with the proximal free end appearing frayed (*long arrow*). The distal free edge is just deep to the laceration (*short arrows*). (*B*) The patient also presented with a painful lump in the palm. Transverse view of the flexor tendons demonstrates the normal echogenic superficial flexor tendon (FDS) overlying the hypoechoic FDP (*asterisk*). The FDP is hypoechoic owing to anisotropy in the retracted bunched-up portion of the torn tendon.

and therefore are more prone to anisotropy and may appear less echogenic than tendons.

Ligament Sprain/Rupture/Avulsion

A spectrum of injuries can result from stress to a ligament. Stretching or impaction on the ligament may lead to a sprain. When the stress exceeds the tensile strength of the ligament, it may rupture or tear. Alternatively, the ligament may remain intact and instead pull off a bony fragment at the attachment site, also known as an avulsion.

Acute sprains of ligaments can demonstrate the following sonographic characteristics: thickening of the ligament, an anechoic region that crosses the ligament, an anechoic band that follows the superficial border of the ligament, or diffuse decreased echogenicity of the ligament (**Fig. 4**A). There may be adjacent blood or fluid and surrounding edema in the subcutaneous tissues.[9]

With a complete ligamentous tear, fluid will extend through the ligament to the subcutaneous surface. With sonography, fluid may be seen surrounding the free edges of the torn ligament. With avulsion injuries, a hyperechoic bone fragment may be seen attached to the bunched up ligament (see **Fig. 4**B). Surrounding fluid or blood may also be detected sonographically.

Lateral Ligament Complex of the Ankle

The most common ligaments to be evaluated in the emergency rooms are those from ankle sprains, and typically involve the lateral collateral ligament complex, which is composed of the anterior talofibular, calcaneofibular, and posterior talofibular ligaments. The anterior talofibular ligament connects the anterior portion of the lateral malleolus with the anterior portion of the talus. The calcaneofibular ligament runs from the inferior portion of the lateral malleolus inferiorly and posteriorly attaching at the calcaneus. Visualization of the calcaneofibular ligament requires dorsiflexion of the foot to stretch out the ligament. The posterior talofibular ligament is difficult to visualize sonographically, coursing from the posterior portion of the lateral malleolus to the posterior portion of the talus. The lateral ligament complex of the ankle can be injured with inversion injuries. In the typical ankle sprain, the only ligament involved is the anterior talofibular ligament. More severe injuries will involve the calcaneofibular ligament, with the most severe involving the posterior tibiofibular ligament.[9] Both the anterior tibiofibular and calcaneofibular ligaments normally measure 2 mm in diameter. Both normally appear hyperechoic; however, the proximal third of the calcaneofibular ligament may appear hypoechoic from obliquity of the ligament. As previously described, an ankle sprain may present sonographically as thickening and decreased echogenicity of the ligament, a tear, or an avulsion.

Ulnar Collateral Ligament Sprain of the Thumb

Another common ligamentous injury involves the ulnar collateral ligament of the first metacarpophalangeal joint, one of the thumb-stabilizing ligaments. Chronic injury has been referred to as "Gamekeeper's thumb," which refers to a laxity in the ulnar collateral ligament. Currently, most injuries have been described in falls that cause an acute abduction injury to the thumb, most often related to skiing, specifically those caused by a ski pole. Ligamentous injury to the ulnar collateral

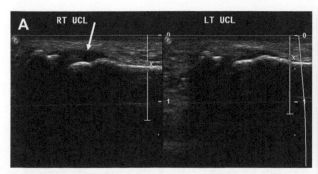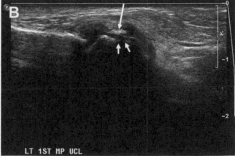

Fig. 4. Gamekeeper's thumb. (*A*) A 36-year-old individual with thumb pain after a ski trip. Comparison long-axis views of the ulnar collateral ligaments (UCL) of the metacarpophalangeal joints of the right and left thumbs show asymmetric thickening of the UCL on the right (*arrow*). The ligament is also decreased in echogenicity when compared with the left. It is difficult to tell whether there is a tear or anisotropy. (*B*) Long-axis view of the UCL in a different patient who experienced acute pain while skiing. The UCL is thickened, heterogeneous, and ill-defined. A bone fragment (*long arrow*) is present, avulsed from the proximal attachment with discontinuity of the underlying cortex (*short arrows*).

ligament can also be associated with an avulsion fracture, typically involving the distal insertion of the ligament on the proximal first carpal.

The ulnar collateral ligament can be visualized sonographically as a compact fibrillary structure extending across the ulnar aspect of the first metacarpophalangeal joint. Dynamic imaging with varus and valgus stress to the thumb can help visualize ligamentous laxity or tear. The bony cortex at the ligamentous attachments should be evaluated for avulsion fractures (see **Fig. 4**B).

MUSCLE

Skeletal muscle is bundled into fascicles. Between 10 and 100 fascicles are contained within a sheath of connective tissue called the perimysium. The fascicles appear hypoechoic and the fascia is hyperechoic. When viewed longitudinally, the perimysium is linearly hyperechoic; when viewed in the transverse dimension, the perimysium appears as diffuse echogenic speckles.

Muscle Tear/Rupture/Contusion

The etiology of acute muscle injury can be either compressive or distractive in nature. Distractive injuries are typically the result of overuse or overstretching, leading to a clinical picture of stiffness and soreness in the muscle region. The most common areas of involvement of muscle injury are the hamstrings, rectus femoris, hip adductor and flexor muscles, and medial gastrocnemius muscle.[10] Distraction injuries most commonly occur at the musculotendinous junction and manifest as partial or complete tears. Sonographic features include disruption and discontinuity of the perimysium and muscle fascicles.

Use of power Doppler can show hypervascularity surrounding a muscle tear. Fluid collections can be seen within the tear. Acute blood appears solid and may mask tears. The treatment is typically conservative, often requiring a more lengthy period of recovery, as additional strain can lead to increased injury. Complete disruption of the entire muscle is often associated with some degree of muscle retraction, usually at the myotendinous junctions. These are typically treated surgically. On ultrasound, complete disruption of the perimysium can be demonstrated with a hyperechoic mass consisting of retracted muscle, with an associated relatively hypoechoic hematoma, referred to as the "clapper in bell" sign.[11]

Compressive injury is usually the result of blunt force trauma. These can result in prolonged soreness in the affected muscle. Hematomas can develop after a compressive injury, which in the acute setting can appear echogenic and solid on ultrasound (**Fig. 5**). With careful scanning, disruption of the normal muscle architecture may be observed. In the subacute setting, the fluid collection will appear heterogeneous, with layering of debris. Eventually, the fluid collection will appear homogeneously hypoechoic to anechoic. Drainage of the homogeneous anechoic fluid collection can result in a faster recovery.[10]

Gastrocnemius Muscle Tear

Another condition that can lead to sudden onset calf pain is a tear of the medial head of the gastrocnemius muscle, another form of "tennis leg." The injury usually results from dorsiflexion of the ankle while the knee is in full extension. On ultrasound, the medial gastrocnemius tapers distally, with the tendon fibers joining with those of the soleus

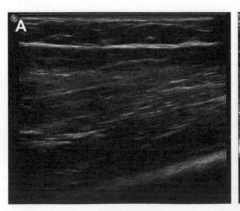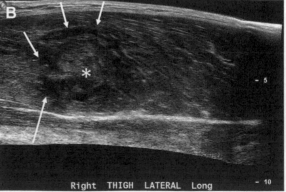

Fig. 5. Muscle injury. (A) Long-axis view of normal muscle. Note the echogenic linear fascia and hypoechoic appearance to muscle fibers. (B) Muscle contusion. Hematoma (*asterisk*) within the rectus femoris muscle after blunt trauma to the thigh. The surrounding muscle architecture is disrupted with displacement of the adjacent muscle fibers (*arrows*).

and lateral gastrocnemius muscle tendons to form the Achilles tendon. The gastrocnemius muscle is more superficial to the soleus muscle. Tears to the medial head of the gastrocnemius muscle typically occur at the musculotendinous junction and appear as a disruption in the normal longitudinal fibrillar pattern with a hypoechoic hematoma sometimes visualized at the site of disruption, which can demonstrate posterior acoustic enhancement (**Fig. 6**A).[4] With severe tears, the fluid can be seen on transverse images extending along the entire length of the medial head of the gastrocnemius, in contradistinction to a plantaris tendon tear, which results in a tubular fluid collection between the gastrocnemius and soleus (see **Fig. 6**B).

Myositis Ossificans

Myositis ossificans is a benign ossifying soft tissue mass located in the muscle. History of trauma is often elicited from patients with myositis ossificans, but other nontraumatic etiologies have been identified. Clinically, myositis ossificans can be asymptomatic or present as pain, swelling, and loss of muscle function that is disproportionate to the degree of trauma. Most ossifying lesions arise in the larger muscle groups of the extremities. The coarse calcification can be seen later on in the development of the lesion, typically 3 to 8 weeks after injury, with calcification starting peripherally and progressing centrally.[12] This can be visualized radiographically. However, the initial few weeks of development of myositis ossificans can be radiographically normal. On ultrasound, the early formation of myositis ossificans can be observed as a hypoechoic mass with sheets of echogenic material.[11] Later on, as the coarse calcification develops, the myositis ossificans will appear echoic with acoustic shadowing (**Fig. 7**).

Muscle Hernias

Muscle can herniate into the subcutaneous fat through fascial defects. These are mostly observed in the lower limbs and can occur from trauma, compartment syndrome, and fascial weakness from perforating vessels.[13] The clinical presentation of muscle hernia is a soft tissue mass in the lower limbs that is increased in size when the affected muscle is contracted and decreased when relaxed. Most are asymptomatic, although pain and cramping involving the herniated region can occur. On ultrasound, the thin surface fascia appears echogenic. Ultrasound features of muscle herniation include disruption or elevation of the fascial plane with herniation of muscle into the subcutaneous tissues (**Fig. 8**). The herniated and adjacent nonherniated muscles appear relatively hypoechoic to the rest of the muscle, most likely secondary to anisotropy and/or atrophy of the herniated muscle.[14] The muscle fibroadipose septa can become narrowed as they exit through the herniation leading to a spoke-like appearance.[13] The dynamic nature of sonography can allow for better visualization of the herniation, as the patient can be asked during scanning to contract the affected muscle.

NERVES

Peripheral nerves can be visualized sonographically. The nerves themselves are composed of hypoechoic fascicles with a hyperechoic epineurium, which is composed of collagen and adipose tissue. They have a rounded or ovoid appearance on transverse views.

Traumatic Neuromas

Nerve injury includes complete transection, crushing injuries, and stretching injuries. With complete transection, one may observe discontinuity of the

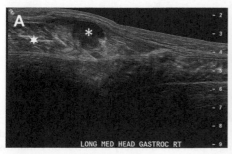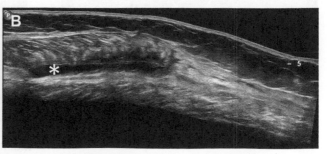

Fig. 6. Gastrocnemius muscle tear. (*A*) Long-axis extended field of view of the medial head of the gastrocnemius muscle (*star*) demonstrates a muscle tear (*asterisk*) with disruption of the muscle fibers and a hematoma within the tear. (*B*) Comparison case of plantaris tendon tear, which can present with similar symptoms. Notice the location of the tubular fluid collection (*asterisk*) deep to the gastrocnemius muscle and just anterior and to the soleus muscle.

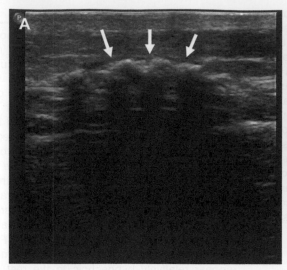
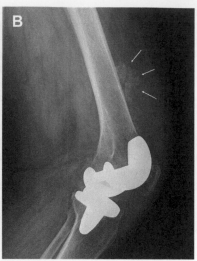

Fig. 7. Myositis ossificans. (*A*) Coarse calcification (*arrows*) is present within the muscle in this long-axis view of the quadriceps muscles. This patient had a history of blunt trauma to the thigh 4 weeks prior. The radiograph was negative. (*B*) Radiograph of the same area obtained 3 weeks later showed calcifications (*arrows*) in the same location.

nerve. A traumatic neuroma may form at the transected end.

Also known as a pseudoneuroma, traumatic neuroma is a non-neoplastic proliferative mass of Schwann cells and nerve cells that occurs at the proximal end of a severed or injured nerve. Clinically, they present as a firm nodule that may be tender or painful to palpation. Sonographically, this appears as hypoechoic fusiform or rounded thickening of the nerve end (**Fig. 9**). Although a neoplastic lesion or focal inflammation in the nerve may have a similar appearance, the history of local trauma helps make the diagnosis. Stretching or compression may result in fusiform or focal thickening of the nerve, which corresponds with the site of trauma and pain.

SUBCUTANEOUS SOFT TISSUES
Foreign Bodies

Foreign bodies in the soft tissues can lead to swelling and chronic pain, and can serve as a nidus for infection. Foreign bodies within soft tissues are often initially evaluated by radiographs. Although radiographs are useful at identifying radiopaque foreign bodies such as glass,[15] pencil lead, and metal, many foreign objects are not radiopaque, such as wood, stone, and plastic.[16] All soft tissue foreign bodies are echogenic on ultrasound. When present, a hypoechoic halo may represent edema, hemorrhage, or, in the more chronic cases, granulation tissue (**Fig. 10**).[17,18] An acoustic shadow may be present depending on the size and surface

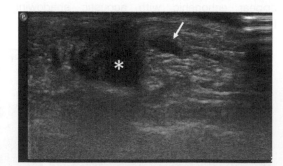

Fig. 8. Muscle hernia. This patient presented with a mass in the shin that increases in size with dorsiflexion of the foot. Long axis scan over the "mass" demonstrates herniation of muscle fibers (*arrows*) through a fascial defect.

Fig. 9. Traumatic neuroma. This patient presented with finger pain and a history of laceration 2 months prior. Scarring related to the laceration is seen presenting as a hypoechoic lesion (*asterisk*). Just proximal to the laceration is focal thickening at the end of the transected nerve (*arrow*). Compression to this area by the transducer reproduced the patient's symptoms.

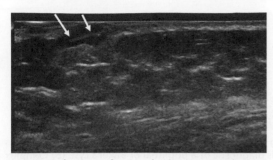

Fig. 10. Soft tissue foreign body. Linear echogenic structure (*arrows*) in the subcutaneous soft tissues corresponds to a wood splinter obtained during a barbecue 2 weeks before presentation. The hypoechoic halo around the splinter is characteristic of granulation reaction around the foreign body that forms over time.

characteristics of the foreign object.[16] Color or power Doppler imaging can demonstrate surrounding hyperemia. Sonography allows for the patient to pinpoint the source of irritation, allowing for a high degree of accuracy in foreign body detection.[19] It can also prove useful in the surgical removal of foreign objects, as it can provide additional information such as depth, size, and important adjacent structures such as vasculature and nerves.

Infection

Cellulitis is an infection of the skin and subcutaneous soft tissues. On ultrasound, this can manifest as a diffuse thickening of the skin and subcutaneous tissues. Anechoic strands of fluid can dissect the fibrous fascia of the subcutaneous fat leading to a cobblestone appearance.[20] This appearance is nonspecific and indistinguishable from other causes of soft tissue edema.

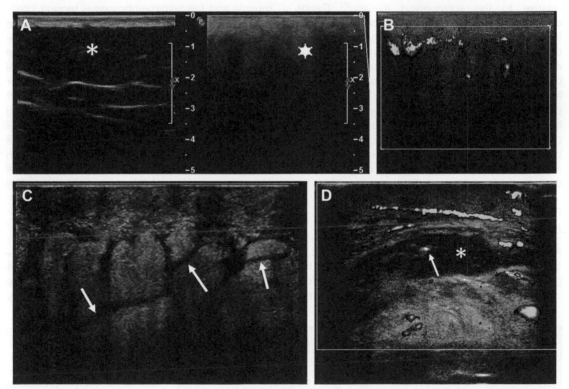

Fig. 11. Soft tissue infections. (*A*) Comparison image of the soft tissues in a patient presenting with left thigh swelling and tenderness. The left image is of the unaffected asymptomatic right thigh. The subcutaneous fat is hypoechoic (*asterisk*) punctuated by echogenic linear retinacula or fascia. The subcutaneous fat of the left thigh is increased in echogenicity (*star*). (*B*) Power Doppler imaging of the same area demonstrates increased vascularity, indicating inflammation. (*C*) Edema may also present as anechoic strands of fluid (*arrows*) dissecting along fascial planes within the subcutaneous fat. (*D*) Transverse power Doppler scan of an amputation stump in a patient presenting with fever, pain, and swelling over the stump. A complex fluid collection (*asterisk*) is present in the symptomatic site, containing punctate echogenic foci (*arrows*) which represent gas bubbles. Notice abnormal increased echogenicity of the surrounding adjacent subcutaneous fat and increased vascularity demonstrated by power Doppler.

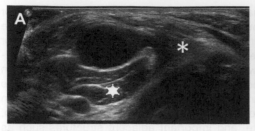
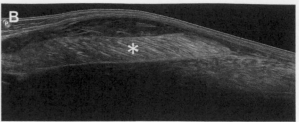

Fig. 12. Ruptured popliteal cyst. (*A*) Fluid collection arising from between the medial head of the gastrocnemius muscle (*star*) and the semimembranosus tendon (*asterisk*) is diagnostic of a popliteal or Baker's cyst. (*B*) Complex fluid extending along the calf located superficial to the gastrocnemius muscle (*asterisk*) is the result of a recent popliteal cyst rupture.

Alternatively, subcutaneous fat, which is typically hypoechoic, may appear more echogenic with diffuse edema. Power Doppler imaging may indicate increased vascularity in the setting of inflammation (**Fig. 11**A–C).

Abscesses are generally hypoechoic, but can have a variable appearance on ultrasound, sometimes appearing as isoechoic or hyperechoic relative to the surrounding tissues.[20] Gentle compression of the abscess can be useful when the abscess is isoechoic or hyperechoic to demonstrate flow of the purulent material.[21] The rim of the abscess can be echogenic. There can be internal septations and punctate echogenic foci, which can reflect debris or gas. Color or power Doppler imaging can show surrounding hyperemia, with lack of flow to the central necrotic core (see **Fig. 10**D).[20] If necessary, a needle can be sonographically guided into the collection to aspirate contents for pathogenic diagnosis and therapy.

BURSA
Ruptured Baker's Cyst

A Baker's cyst, also known as a popliteal cyst, is a benign posterior outpouching of the gastrocnemius-semimembranosus bursa. Most of the "cysts" retain their communication with the

synovial sac of the knee joint and are therefore not true cysts. Large Baker's cysts are palpable and can rupture, leading to acute calf pain and swelling, mimicking other pathologies, such as a deep venous thrombosis or traumatic injury.

On ultrasound, a Baker's cyst appears as a fluid collection in the popliteal fossa extending from between the medial head of the gastrocnemius muscle and the semimembranosus tendon inferiorly into the calf (**Fig. 12**A). The fluid may be anechoic when noted in patients with noninflammatory knee arthritis but can also contain internal echoes in the presence of blood or debris, as may seen the setting of trauma, infection, or inflammatory arthritis. A ruptured Baker's cyst will show simple or complicated fluid tracking medially within the subcutaneous tissues of the calf superficial to the gastrocnemius muscle (see **Fig. 12**B) in contradistinction to the fluid collection in a plantaris tendon tear, which will accumulate between the soleus and gastrocnemius muscles (see **Fig. 6**B).[4]

JOINTS
Effusions and Septic Arthritis

Septic arthritis is an infection involving the joint space that can lead to rapid destruction of the joint. Establishment of a diagnosis is made by

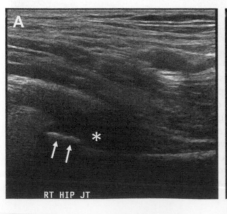
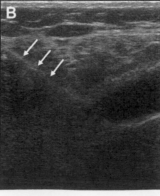

Fig. 13. Joint effusion. (*A*) Long axis view of the femoral neck demonstrates fluid (*asterisk*) corresponding to a joint effusion in this patient presenting with hip pain and fever 3 weeks after hip replacement surgery. The hardware is indicated by the arrows. (*B*) Ultrasound can be used to guide a needle (*arrows*) into the fluid to confirm the diagnosis of infection.

arthrocentesis, and this has traditionally been performed using external landmarks or under fluoroscopic guidance. However, overlying soft tissue infections can sometimes mimic a joint effusion. In the setting of a clinically suspected but absent joint effusion, an arthrocentesis through an overlying soft tissue infection can introduce infection into a previously sterile joint space.[22] Sonography can play a role in distinguishing between a soft tissue infection and an effusion, as sonography is sensitive in detecting effusions, particularly in the knee, wrist, and elbow (**Fig. 13**A).[20] Ultrasound can also be used to guide a needle for fluid aspiration (see **Fig. 13**B). Color Doppler can be used to avoid vascular structures during an arthrocentesis. However, ultrasound does not distinguish between septic and aseptic effusions, and an arthrocentesis is required to make a diagnosis.

BONES
Fractures

Although not considered the first line in imaging for fractures, in remote locations or trauma settings where radiography is not available, sonography may provide an alternative modality for evaluation.

Although the highly reflective and absorptive nature of bone limits evaluation of the deep bony structures, ultrasound does have utility in evaluating the contour of soft tissue bony interface and the bony surfaces. This allows for pathology such as fractures to be visualized on ultrasound. A fracture can be identified by ultrasound as

a discontinuity or step-off of the cortex (**Fig. 14**), or by an angular buckling of the cortex. Associated findings include subperiosteal hematoma with overlying soft tissue edema.[23] Localization of pain by the patient can help guide sonographic detection of radiographically occult fractures. Fractures can also be followed by ultrasound. The initial hypoechoic fracture line will be replaced over time by hyperechoic periosteal reaction that bridges the fractured gap, which will demonstrate increased shadowing as the healing progresses.[23]

Although ultrasound cannot replace radiography in the evaluation of fractures, it can provide useful information about concomitant soft tissue involvement and can serve as an adjunct in evaluating adjacent vascular structures for injury.

SUMMARY

Ultrasound is extremely well suited to evaluating the extremities in patients who have been injured. It can also be used in other emergency department situations, such as to evaluate acutely painful conditions, including fluid collections, infections, and foreign bodies.

In situations where conventional radiography is not available, including trauma scenes and mass-casualty situations, or at the bedside in the setting of unstable trauma, the decreasing size and cost of portable sonographic equipment make it a first-line choice for evaluation of the extremities.

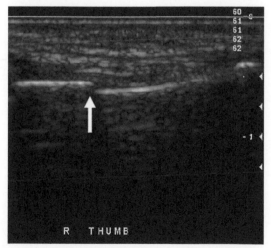

Fig. 14. Fracture. Long axis view of the proximal phalanx of the left first digit demonstrates cortical discontinuity (*arrow*) compatible with a fracture. This was radiographically occult. The patient presented to the ultrasound department owing to persistent pain after dropping a heavy object on the first digit.

REFERENCES

1. Lee JC, Healy JC. Normal sonographic anatomy of the wrist and hand. Radiographics 2005;25:1577–90.
2. Robinson P. Sonography of common tendon injuries. Am J Roentgenol 2009;193:607–18.
3. Hartgerink P, Fessell DP, Jacobson JA, et al. Full-versus partial-thickness Achilles tendon tears: sonographic accuracy and characterization in 26 cases with surgical correlation. Radiology 2001;220:406–12.
4. Jamadar DA, Jacobson JA, Theisen SE, et al. Sonography of the painful calf: differential considerations. Am J Roentgenol 2002;179:706–16.
5. Khan KM, Cook JL, Bonar F, et al. Histopathology of common overuse tendon conditions: update and implications for clinical management. Sports Med 1999;27(6):393–408.
6. Carr JC, Hanly S, Griffin J, et al. Sonography of the patellar tendon and adjacent structures in pediatric and adult patients. Am J Roentgenol 2001;176:1535–9.
7. Martinoli C, Bianchi S, Prato N, et al. US of the shoulder: non-rotator cuff disorders. Radiographics 2003;23:381–401.

8. Jacobson JA. Fundamentals of musculoskeletal ultrasound. Philadelphia: Saunders; 2007.

9. Peetrons P. Sonography of ankle ligaments. J Clin Ultrasound 2004;32(9):491–9.

10. Middleton WD, Kurtz AB, Hertzberg BS, editors. Ultrasound: the requisites. 2nd edition. St. Louis (MO): Mosby; 2004.

11. Lee JC, Healy JC. Sonography of lower limb muscle injury. Am J Roentgenol 2004;182:341–51.

12. Crundwell N, O'Donnell P, Saifuddin A. Non-neoplastic conditions presenting as soft-tissue tumors. Clin Radiol 2006;62(1):18–27.

13. Beggs I. Sonography of muscle hernias. Am J Roentgenol 2003;180:395–9.

14. van Holsbeeck MT, Introcaso JH, editors. Musculoskeletal ultrasound. 2nd edition. St Louis (MO): Mosby; 2001. p. 64–6.

15. Felman AH, Fisher MS. The radiographic detection of glass in soft tissue. Radiology 1969;92(7):1529–31.

16. Horton LK, Jacobson JA, Powell A, et al. Sonography and radiography of soft-tissue foreign bodies. Am J Roentgenol 2001;176:1155–9.

17. Fornage BD, Schernberg FL. Sonographic diagnosis of foreign bodies of the distal extremities. Am J Roentgenol 1986;147(3):567–9.

18. Jacobson JA, Powell A, Craig JG, et al. Wooden foreign bodies in soft tissue: detection at US. Radiology 1998;206:45–8.

19. Jamadar DA, Jacobson JA, Caoili EM, et al. Musculoskeletal sonography technique: focused versus comprehensive evaluation. Am J Roentgenol 2008; 190:5–9.

20. Bureau NJ, Chhem RK, Cardinal E. Musculoskeletal infections: US manifestations. Radiographics 1999; 19:1585–92.

21. Loyer EM, DuBrow RA, David CL, et al. Imaging of superficial soft-tissue infections: sonographic findings in cases of cellulitis and abscess. Am J Roentgenol 1996;166(1):149–52.

22. Fessell DP, Jacobson JA, Craig J, et al. Using sonography to reveal and aspirate joint effusions. Am J Roentgenol 2000;174:1353–62.

23. Cho KH, Lee YH, Lee SM, et al. Sonography of bone and bone-related diseases of the extremities. J Clin Ultrasound 2004;32(9):511–21.

Sonography Assessment of Acute Ocular Pathology

Megan Leo, MD*, Kristin Carmody, MD, RDMS

KEYWORDS

- Ocular • Hemorrhage • Detachment • Dislocation

BACKGROUND AND INDICATIONS

Ocular complaints comprise an estimated 3% of all emergency department patient visits annually in the United States.[1,2] The use of sonographic examination of the eye in this capacity has been well described in the literature and continues to increase in scope.[3–5] The eye is a fluid-filled structure, providing an ideal acoustic window for sonographic assessment of the intraocular and adjacent structures. Sonography has become a useful adjunct to the traditional evaluation of ocular complaints because it may provide additional information that is not apparent on physical examination and that can help to readily identify disorders and expedite treatment. Emergency physicians have been shown to accurately recognize various ocular disorders with ultrasound compared with other modalities, such as computed tomography (CT) scan of the orbits.[2]

As with many focused ultrasound examinations performed in the acute setting, bedside ocular sonography is meant to be a tailored examination and is therefore limited in scope. The main goal of ocular ultrasound is to identify conditions that require immediate intervention and/or threaten a patient's vision. Ocular sonography can be useful in both traumatic injuries to the orbit and head as well as in the evaluation of nontraumatic eye complaints. Sonographic ultrasound evaluation of the orbit is particularly helpful in patients in whom the physical and fundoscopic examination is limited because of pain and swelling or if the patient's eyelids cannot be sufficiently opened

(**Fig. 1**). Sonographic assessment may also be able to diagnose injuries in the posterior segment of the eye, such as a vitreous hemorrhage, retinal or vitreous detachments,[6,7] lens dislocation, or intraocular foreign body that may be obscured in the setting of corneal swelling or anterior chamber hemorrhage, a condition known as hyphema. For trauma, ultrasound has been shown to be accurate in evaluating extraocular eye movements that may be difficult to assess in the presence of swelling. In addition, ultrasound can be used to evaluate for the pupillary light reflex in a swollen eye. The injured eye is imaged with ultrasound and constriction of the pupil can be observed while shining a light in the contralateral, unaffected eye.[8] In the case of head trauma, ocular sonography can aid in the rapid diagnosis of increased intracranial pressure by detecting an increase in the optic nerve sheath diameter (ONSD).[9–11] Bedside ocular ultrasound is also useful in evaluating patients with nontraumatic conditions that require emergent treatment, such as central retinal artery or vein occlusion.

NORMAL OCULAR ANATOMY
Landmarks

The sonographic landmarks of the eye are the lens, posterior wall of the globe, and the optic nerve. Other visible anatomy includes the orbital bone, the cornea, the iris, the pupil, the anterior chamber, and vitreous body (**Fig. 2**). It is important to identify these structures at the beginning of the examination, especially in the setting of massive trauma,

No financial disclosures.
Department of Emergency Medicine, Boston University Medical School, Boston Medical Center, One Boston Medical Center Place, Dowling One South, Boston, MA 02118, USA
* Corresponding author.
E-mail address: megan.leo@bmc.org

Ultrasound Clin 6 (2011) 227–234
doi:10.1016/j.cult.2011.03.002
1556-858X/11/$ – see front matter © 2011 Elsevier Inc. All rights reserved.

ultrasound.theclinics.com

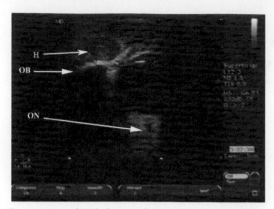

Fig. 1. Periorbital hemorrhage (H) and swelling impeded physical and fundoscopic eye examination in this patient who suffered blunt trauma. Sonography allowed assessment of the orbital structures, including normal orbital bone (OB) and optic nerve posteriorly (ON). (*Courtesy of* Andreas Dewitz, MD, RDMS, Boston Medical Center.)

in which injuries such as lens dislocation or globe rupture can distort the normal eye anatomy.

Orbital Bone

The orbital bones surround the globe and appear hyperechoic with posterior acoustic shadowing on ultrasound, similar to other bony structures that impede the ultrasound beam and create an artifact posteriorly. The orbital bones should have a smooth, sharp edge (see **Figs. 1** and **2**) and any disruption may suggest an orbital fracture.

Anterior Chamber

The anterior chamber is a fluid-filled structure that is bounded by the iris and cornea and appears black or anechoic on ultrasound because of its simple fluid contents. The cornea is the first structure visualized on ultrasound because it sits most anteriorly and protects the iris, pupil, and anterior chamber. The cornea appears as a convex, thin, echogenic stripe overlying the anterior eye (see **Fig. 2**). The most common pathologies encountered in the anterior chamber include hyphema and glaucoma. Although sonographic evaluation of the fine details of the anterior chamber require specialized high-frequency probes, typically more than 20 MHz, an appreciation for disrupted normal anatomy may be possible during the focused bedside ocular examination with standard probes.

Posterior Chamber

The posterior chamber is a small area that exists between the iris and the lens. It is also fluid filled, and so appears anechoic on ultrasound. The pupil

can be visualized as an oblong structure sitting in the center of the iris just anterior to the lens (see **Fig. 2**).

Lens

The lens is a biconvex hyperechoic structure that sits behind the pupil and iris, attached peripherally by the ciliary body (see **Fig. 2**). It helps to refract light that gets focused onto the retina. A normal lens creates reverberation artifact, seen as linear, repetitive, hyperechoic lines emanating from its posterior surface.

Vitreous Body

The vitreous body is located between the lens and the posterior wall of the eye. It is normally anechoic, or black, on ultrasound and is filled with vitreous humor (see **Fig. 2**).

Retina

The retina comprises the posterior wall of the eye and is normally adherent to the sclera (see **Fig. 2**). It appears as a smooth line without disruption outlining the posterior wall of the globe. The retina is usually not clearly delineated from the other choroidal layers on ultrasound unless it is disrupted.

Posterior Structures

The structures posterior to the globe that can be seen easily by sonography include the optic nerve and sheath and the retrobulbar space. The blood supply to the eye is primarily from the ophthalmic artery, which gives off its first branch, the central retinal artery. The central retinal artery and vein can be identified within the optic nerve sheath using color flow Doppler (**Fig. 3**).

Spectral Doppler can be used to obtain waveforms that depict the flow velocity within the blood vessels. These waveforms can be used to differentiate arterial from venous blood flow (**Fig. 4**).

The optic nerve appears hypoechoic and extends posterior to the globe, whereas the sheath surrounding the nerve is hyperechoic. The ONSD can be measured 3 mm posterior from the retina and across its short axis to evaluate for increased intracranial pressure (see **Fig. 2**; **Fig. 5**).

ULTRASOUND TECHNIQUE

Because the eye is a superficial structure, imaging is best accomplished by using a high-frequency linear probe, with a minimum frequency of 7.5 MHz, noting that resolution improves with higher-frequency probes.

The settings should be optimized for maximal resolution, particularly in the near field. Many

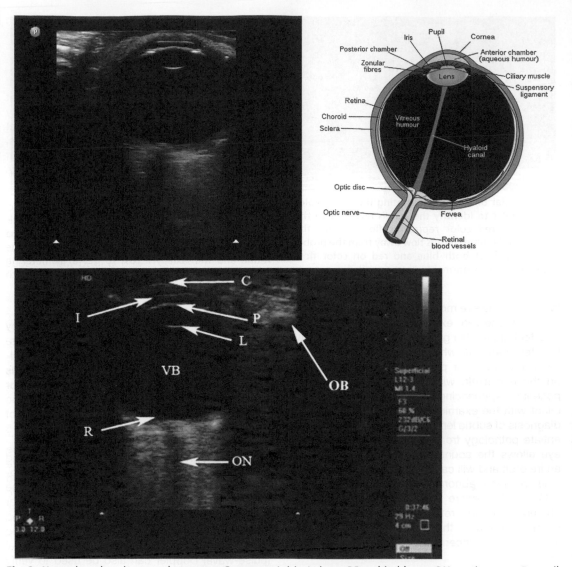

Fig. 2. Normal ocular ultrasound anatomy. C, cornea; I, iris; L, lens; OB, orbital bone; ON, optic nerve; P, pupil; R, retina; VB, vitreous body.

manufactures have provided an ocular, superficial, or small-parts preset that can be used and adjusted as needed.

As with any ultrasound application, acoustic coupling gel is an important medium, needed to reduce artifacts and produce sharper images. A barrier should be placed over the closed eye, if available, to prevent irritation or infection, and this can be accomplished by using a Tegaderm (3M Company) or a similar thin barrier.

Imaging Protocol

Imaging of the eye should be performed in 2 planes to ensure a complete evaluation of the orbit and adjacent structures. Scanning should begin in the

transverse plane across the eyelid and the key landmarks of the lens, posterior structures, and optic nerve should be identified to confirm a midline scan. The probe should then be rocked superiorly and inferiorly to fan completely through the whole orbit. This allows for a complete interrogation of the eye and all of its structures. After adequate transverse images are obtained, the probe should be turned 90° into a sagittal position and the probe rocked medially and laterally to once again fully evaluate all structures. The unaffected eye should also be scanned for comparison.

An alternative technique is for the operator to keep the probe static over the midline position of the eye and have patients move their eyeball while the lid is shut. This technique allows the operator

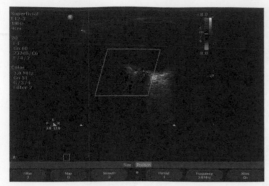

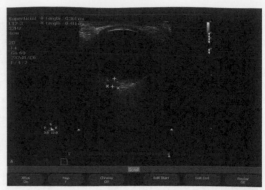

Fig. 3. Ocular ultrasound illustrating the use of color flow Doppler to identify the vessels posterior to the retina. The red color represents flow toward the probe and the blue color is flow away from the probe. The presence of both blue and red on color flow Doppler suggests normal bidirectional flow.

Fig. 5. The optic nerve appears as an anechoic structure extending posteriorly from the retina. The optic sheath is hyperechoic and surrounds the nerve. The sheath should be measured 3 mm back from the retina and transaxially across to get a diameter. In the image above, the ONSD measures 4.1 mm, which is within normal limits.

to observe the eye moving in all 4 quadrants, confirming preserved extraocular muscle function. This technique also gives the examiner the ability to interrogate the whole orbit without having to move the probe or place unnecessary pressure on the eye itself, which is beneficial when the patient is experiencing discomfort and is noncompliant with the examination. It can also aid in the diagnosis of subtle lens subluxations and to differentiate pathology from artifact. Movement of the eye allows the sound beam to fan through the entire orbit and will cause an artifact to disappear, whereas a true abnormality will remain.

Once the entire globe, including anterior chamber, vitreous, retina, and posterior orbit, has been interrogated, the ONSD may be measured if there is a concern for increased intracranial

pressure. This measurement is accomplished by obtaining a midline image of the globe in the transverse axis, so that the optic nerve is clearly visualized running posterior to the retina. The image is frozen and a measurement is made 3 mm posterior to the retina along the parallel axis of the optic nerve. Then a short axis measurement is taken of the nerve sheath. Any measurement more than 5 mm is considered abnormal (see **Fig. 5**; **Fig. 6**).

If a patient presents with sudden vision loss and there is a concern for arterial or venous compromise, ultrasound can be used to evaluate the central retinal arteries and veins. The vascular plexus is located behind the posterior wall and color flow Doppler can be used to assess for the presence of flow (see **Fig. 3**). In addition spectral (pulse-wave) Doppler can also be used to verify

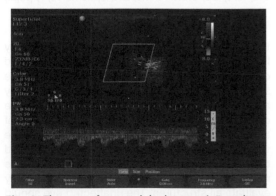

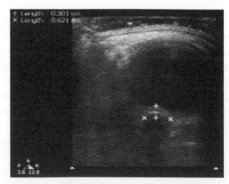

Fig. 4. The use of spectral (pulse-wave) Doppler to identify central retinal artery and central retinal vein blood flow. The tracing at the bottom of the screen depicts velocity over time, with venous flow depicted above the baseline and arterial flow depicted below the baseline.

Fig. 6. Ocular ultrasound illustrating a widened optic nerve sheath. This patient had increased intracranial pressure from pseudotumor cerebri and had an optic nerve sheath measurement of 6.2 mm, as depicted in the upper left corner of the image.

arterial and venous waveforms and their relative velocities (see **Fig. 4**). Specific velocity measurements to diagnose central venous and arterial occlusions are usually beyond the scope of emergency medicine practice, but, if an obvious decrease in blood flow is detected, ophthalmology should be contacted immediately.

OCULAR PATHOLOGY

1. Lens dislocation or subluxation is most often caused by blunt trauma to the orbit. It occurs when the zonular fibers that hold the lens in place are disrupted.[12] The lens appears as an oval echogenic structure that lies posterior to the ciliary body and normally has many reverberation artifacts. A complete lens dislocation can be obvious on ultrasound because the lens is seen remote from its usual position behind the pupil and is often suspended within the vitreous body of the posterior orbit (**Fig. 7**).

   Lens subluxation (partial dislocation) can be much more difficult to diagnose because there are only slight changes in the position of the lens. A subluxed lens may be detected on ultrasound by asking patients to move their eyes during the examination. A normal lens moves in concordance with the other orbital structures, whereas a subluxed lens may appear to move out of position behind the iris.[1] A comparison with the contralateral eye should always be done to evaluate for symmetry.

2. Hyphema is the occurrence of blood in the anterior chamber and is typically associated with an acute increase in intraocular pressure. It is most often caused by blunt trauma but can also occur in the presence of abnormal vessels in the eye caused by diabetes, chronic inflammation, surgery, or malignancy. Depending on the degree of the hyphema, the patient may have no visual changes or, as in the case of complete hyphema, may have light perception only.[12] Although hyphema is usually a clinical diagnosis, ultrasound can aid in the diagnosis when periorbital swelling prevents a complete examination of the anterior chamber. Sonographically, a hyphema appears as a hyperechoic layering in the anterior chamber.

3. Globe rupture may occur in the setting of blunt or penetrating trauma. If globe rupture is suspected, an ocular ultrasound should not be performed because of the risk of further injury to the eye from inadvertent pressure from the application of the ultrasound probe. It is important to know how to recognize a ruptured globe because, once this is seen on ultrasound, the examination should be stopped to prevent further injury. Globe rupture can be detected on an ultrasound examination by noting a collapsed anterior chamber, an asymmetric posterior chamber, or scleral fold.[3,5] There is often an associated hemorrhage (**Fig. 8**).

4. Vitreous hemorrhage is the extravasation of blood into the spaces formed within and around the vitreous body. It may occur because of blunt trauma and direct retinal tear or from any condition that causes neovascularization, including diabetes.[12] This bleeding can result in acute visual changes depending on the amount of opaque blood within the vitreous. On ultrasound, a vitreous hemorrhage appears as a bright echogenic layer within the posterior eye (**Fig. 9**). If the vitreous hemorrhage is large enough, as sometimes seen with blunt trauma, the entire body can be obscured (see **Fig. 8**).

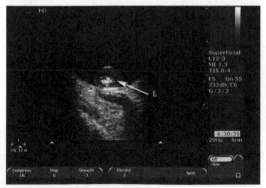

Fig. 7. A posterior lens dislocation. Note the hyperechoic lens floating in the vitreous body in the posterior eye (*arrow*). (*Courtesy of* Andreas Dewitz, MD, RDMS, Boston Medical Center.)

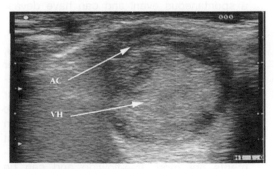

Fig. 8. A globe rupture with vitreous hemorrhage (VH). Note the collapsed anterior chamber (AC) and misshapen posterior chamber of the orbit. The vitreous hemorrhage appears as the hyperechoic material filling the whole globe. (*Courtesy of* Andreas Dewitz, MD, RDMS, Boston Medical Center.)

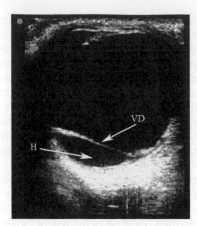

Fig. 9. Vitreous detachment and hemorrhage. The detachment (VD) is seen as a bright echogenic line in the posterior chamber. The hemorrhage (H) appears as a murky hyperechoic material posterior to the detachment. (*Courtesy of* Andreas Dewitz, MD, RDMS, Boston Medical Center.)

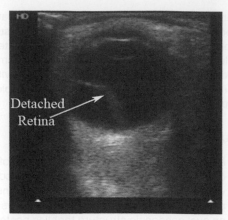

Fig. 10. An ocular ultrasound illustrating a retinal detachment. Note its hyperechoic, free-floating appearance within the vitreous body.

5. Vitreous detachment occurs when the vitreous body becomes detached from the retina. This detachment may occur in the setting of trauma, after surgery, or spontaneously over time as the vitreous peels away from the retina in older patients. Patients often describe floaters or shadows in their field of vision. Sonographically, it is typically seen as a V-shaped line within the vitreous and does not float with eye movement.[3] There is often a vitreous hemorrhage associated with it (see **Fig. 9**).

6. Retinal detachment occurs when the retina peels away from its support tissue along the posterior wall of the orbit. Patients describe symptoms that are similar to vitreous detachment, and can also describe flashing lights. Detachments can result from trauma or a spontaneous event and can have devastating consequences if not diagnosed early.[3] Small retinal tears can be seen as slight, hyperechoic, linear protrusions into the vitreous, or may be as subtle as subretinal fluid. Larger retinal detachments can be seen as hyperechoic lines within the vitreous that appear mobile with eye movements when they are acute (**Fig. 10**). Vitreous detachments often appear as V-shaped lines that are adherent to the posterior wall, whereas retinal detachments are more free-flowing and can be seen extending farther into the center of the globe when imaged on ultrasound.

7. Intraocular foreign body (IOFB) may also present as pain and acute visual changes. An IOFB may be present within the cornea, vitreous, retina, or surrounding soft tissue, and therefore the orbit must be scanned thoroughly. In the case of penetrating trauma, the foreign body is often within the vitreous (**Fig. 11**).

Although CT scan remains the gold standard for identifying IOFB, ultrasound may help to locate IOFBs that are radiolucent on CT. Depending on the composition of the IOFB, it may have varying degrees of echogenicity. There is often a shadowing effect that occurs when the ultrasound waves are unable to penetrate a solid object (see **Fig. 11**). This effect appears as a hypoechoic or anechoic

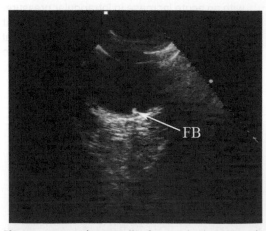

Fig. 11. Intraocular metallic foreign body (FB) in the posterior eye. Note its hyperechoic appearance and the posterior shadowing produced as a black anechoic line extending posteriorly behind the orbit. This artifact is caused by the impedance of the ultrasound beam by the foreign object. (*Courtesy of* Andreas Dewitz, MD, RDMS, Boston Medical Center.)

signal posterior to the object. Metallic foreign bodies are very hyperechoic and, in addition to a shadowing effect, often produce various known artifacts such as reverberation and ring-down artifacts. Color Doppler can also be used to better identify a foreign body that is highly reflective by producing a characteristic twinkling artifact. This artifact is seen as a rapidly alternating mixture of red and blue off a highly reflective foreign body with a rough surface.[13]

8. Retrobulbar hematoma is usually the result of significant blunt trauma to the orbit. There is often periorbital swelling associated with it, making the use of ultrasound especially helpful for the diagnosis. The hematoma has a black or anechoic appearance just posterior to the globe. The posterior aspect of the eye may also be distorted because of the pressure created by the traumatic hematoma pushing on the globe.[3,5]

9. Central retinal artery or vein occlusion can present as a painless, sudden loss of vision. Color Doppler placed posterior to the globe, where the vessels enter, can be used to identify the presence of blood flow (see **Fig. 3**).[14] Absence of bidirectional flow suggests vascular occlusion and disorders. Spectral Doppler can be used to confirm both the presence of venous and arterial waveforms (see **Fig. 4**).

10. ONSD measured by bedside ultrasound has been shown to correlate with both CT findings of increased intracranial pressure and invasive intracranial monitoring.[9–11] ONSD should be measured with the globe in midline position so that the optic nerve is clearly visualized running posterior to the retina. After freezing the image, a measurement is made 3 mm posterior to the retina along the parallel axis of the optic nerve, and then a short axis measurement is taken of the nerve sheath. Any measurement more than 5 mm is considered abnormal (see **Figs. 5** and **6**). To get the most accurate measurement, the ONSD should be calculated by measuring the optic nerve sheath in both the short and long axis bilaterally, and the average of all 4 measurements should be taken. The ONSD should not replace other imaging studies for evaluation of increased intracranial pressure, but may serve as an adjunct in the initial evaluation.

11. Papilledema may also be seen on ultrasound in the setting of increased intracranial pressure.[9] This is seen as a protrusion of the optic disc from the retina.

SUMMARY

Bedside ocular sonography continues to have a growing role in the acute care setting. The main objective of this bedside examination is to determine which patients require immediate ophthalmology consultation and treatment. The use of ocular sonography in the emergency department can expedite the diagnosis and treatment of patients with visual complaints. It provides a rapid assessment of the eye with minimal discomfort to the patient and without radiation exposure.

Ultrasound is ideal in the trauma patient who has extensive periorbital swelling or injury. It can provide additional information when patients cannot cooperate with a fundoscopic examination or for evaluation of the globe when severe edema, chemosis, or hyphemas are present. Ultrasound is also helpful when evaluating unstable patients who cannot go for imaging outside the emergency department or intensive care unit.

Ocular ultrasound should be used in conjunction with a thorough eye examination and is not meant to replace more sensitive radiological tests. It is the perfect adjunct to use in combination with a thorough history and eye examination and can serve as an important screening tool in dangerous ocular conditions.

REFERENCES

1. Rosen P, editor. Emergency medicine concepts and clinical practice. 4th edition. St Louis (MO): Mosby; 1997. p. 2243–5.

2. Blaivas M, Theodoro D, Sierzenski PR. A study of bedside ocular ultrasonography in the emergency department. Acad Emerg Med 2002;9(8):791–9.

3. John Ma O, Mateer J, Blaivas M. Emergency ultrasound. 2nd edition. New York (NY): McGraw-Hill; 2008. p. 449–62.

4. Price DD, Simon BC, Park RS. Evolution of emergency ultrasound. Cal J Emerg Med 2003;4(4):82–8.

5. Blaivas M. Bedside emergency department ultrasonography in the evaluation of ocular pathology. Acad Emerg Med 2000;7:947–50.

6. Yoonessi R, Hussain A, Jang TB. Bedside ocular ultrasound for the detection of retinal detachment in the emergency department. Acad Emerg Med 2010;17(9):913–7.

7. Shinar Z, Chan L, Orlinsky M. Use of ocular ultrasound for the evaluation of retinal detachment. J Emerg Med 2011;40(1):53–7.

8. Harries A, Shah S, Teismann N, et al. Ultrasound assessment of extraocular movements and pupillary light reflex in ocular trauma. Am J Emerg Med 2010; 28(8):956–9.

9. Blaivas M, Theodoro D, Sierzenski PR. Elevated intracranial pressure detected by bedside emergency ultrasonography of the optic nerve sheath. Acad Emerg Med 2003;10(4):376–81.

10. Tayal VS, Neulander M, Norton HJ, et al. Emergency department sonographic measurement of optic nerve sheath diameter to detect findings of increased intracranial pressure in adult head injury patients. Ann Emerg Med 2007;49(4):508–14.

11. Kimberly HH, Shah S, Marill K, et al. Correlation of optic nerve sheath diameter with direct measurement

of intracranial pressure. Acad Emerg Med 2008;15(2): 201–4.

12. Bradford CA. Basic ophthalmology. 7th edition. San Francisco (CA): American Academy of Ophthalmology; 1999.

13. Ustymowicz A, Krejza J, Mariak Z. Twinkling artifact in color Doppler imaging of the orbit. J Ultrasound Med 2002;21(5):559–63.

14. Dimitrova G, Kato S. Color Doppler imaging of retinal diseases [review]. Surv Ophthalmol 2010; 55(3):193–214.

Ultrasound in the Critically Ill

Mark W. Byrne, MD*, James Q. Hwang, MD, RDMS, RDCS

KEYWORDS

• Ultrasound • Shock • Critically ill patients

The critically ill patient in extremis presents one of the greatest challenges to emergency providers and intensivists. Upon arrival to the emergency department (ED) or intensive care unit (ICU), little may be known about the patient's underlying medical conditions or the events that led up to the present situation. Critically ill patients often are unable to provide a meaningful history, due to severe dyspnea, pain, or alterations in consciousness. Vital signs and the physical exam become essential in guiding patient management, but findings are often nonspecific and can overlap significantly among various etiologies of shock. Such patients are frequently hemodynamically unstable, and empiric resuscitation must be started at the same time the initial diagnostic evaluation is being performed. The urgency of the patient's condition may dictate initiation of key therapeutic interventions prior to confirmatory laboratory testing or consultative diagnostic imaging.

There exists the need for a rapid and immediately available means to evaluate patients in extremis. Ultrasound, performed by the clinician sonographer directly at the bedside of an unstable patient, has been proposed as just such a tool. A sonographic assessment of critically ill patients provides valuable information that can guide the clinician during the initial evaluation and stabilization of undifferentiated shock. This article seeks to demonstrate how point-of-care ultrasound may be used to rapidly assess the underlying physiology leading to a patient's shock state; to identify potentially lethal, yet reversible, conditions that otherwise may not be readily diagnosed at the bedside; and to guide resuscitation, in particular as it relates to volume status. Previous applications of emergency ultrasound have focused on visualizing disease pathology and providing guidance for procedures. Representing a departure from such traditional uses, the proposed ultrasound evaluation seeks to assess the underlying physiology in critically ill patients and to follow how it evolves in real time in response to resuscitative interventions.

LIMITATIONS IN CURRENT PRACTICE

A typical sequence of events occurs in the hospital setting after a patient presents to the ED or ICU. The patient is evaluated by the clinician; additional diagnostic imaging, consisting of radiography, computed tomography (CT), ultrasound, or echocardiography, is ordered by the clinician; the diagnostic study is performed by a technician, usually only after the patient has been transferred outside the department to the radiology, vascular, or echocardiography suite; images are transferred to and subsequently interpreted by the radiologist or cardiologist; and interpretations are relayed to the managing clinician, who then uses this information to make clinical decisions regarding patient care.

While this sequence of events may work satisfactorily for patients in an outpatient setting and clinically stable patients in the ED or ICU, it may lead to significant treatment delays in critically ill patients who present in extremis. For hemodynamically unstable patients, treatment frequently must be initiated immediately on arrival, and care plans cannot be delayed while awaiting performance and interpretation of consultative studies. Critically ill patients in the ED and ICU are often

Department of Emergency Medicine, Brigham & Women's Hospital, Neville House, 75 Francis Street, Boston, MA 02115, USA
* Corresponding author.
E-mail address: mwbyrne.md@gmail.com

Ultrasound Clin 6 (2011) 235–259
doi:10.1016/j.cult.2011.03.003
1556-858X/11/$ – see front matter © 2011 Published by Elsevier Inc.

too unstable to leave monitored patient care areas, and portable studies using moveable equipment, whether they are radiographs, ultrasound, or echocardiograms, must be performed by the consultative services. Many of these consultative services may be unavailable during evening and overnight hours, in particular in community hospital settings; however, critically ill patients present to the hospital irrespective of time of day.

Point-of-care ultrasound strives to improve patient care by diagnosing conditions earlier in a patient's course, especially when those conditions are potentially lethal and treatment is time sensitive. The utility of ultrasound to evaluate patients presenting with acute trauma[1–3] and for guidance in emergent procedures[4–7] has been validated in the literature and is now well accepted in the medical community. The American College of Surgeons has incorporated the Focused Assessment with Sonography in Trauma (FAST) exam into their Advanced Trauma Life Support (ATLS) protocol,[8] and the Agency for Healthcare Research and Quality (AHRQ) included ultrasound-guided vascular access as one of its recommended patient safety practices.[9] Other focused ultrasound applications have been validated for performance at the patient bedside, including assessment of the aorta to exclude abdominal aortic aneurysm (AAA)[10,11] and limited bedside echocardiography.[12,13] The American Society of Echocardiography (ASE), in a consensus statement with the American College of Emergency Physicians (ACEP), recently acknowledged the role of focused cardiac ultrasound (FOCUS) in the emergent setting.[14] Applications traditionally thought not amenable to ultrasound, such as assessment of the lungs, have been developed by clinician sonographers and are expanding in scope and utility.[15,16] In addition, applications previously established by other specialties, such as measurement of the inferior vena cava (IVC) for volume status,[17,18] are being integrated into point-of-care ultrasound evaluations in the ED and ICU.

CATEGORIES OF SHOCK

Shock is defined as a state of inadequate perfusion to bodily tissues. Hypotensive blood pressures are characteristic, although not necessarily present, in patients with shock. There are 4 main categories of shock: cardiogenic, hypovolemic, distributive, and obstructive (**Fig. 1**). Cardiogenic shock frequently results from left ventricle (LV) failure; however, it may also originate from arrhythmias, such as ventricular tachycardia; acute valvular insufficiency, such as failure of the posterior leaflet of the mitral valve in the setting of an inferior myocardial infarction; or right ventricle (RV) failure from a right-sided infarction. Hypovolemic shock, a state of severe intravascular volume depletion, may result from a variety of causes. Occult hemorrhage, as from gastrointestinal bleeding or ruptured AAA, as well as severe dehydration, such as in hyperosmolar nonketotic coma, are common causes in the medical patient. Distributive shock results from vasodilation or leakage of intravascular fluid and most commonly results from infectious (septic) or inflammatory (third-spacing) causes in the ED and ICU setting. Although less common, distributive shock can also result from anaphylactic and neurogenic etiologies. Obstructive shock occurs when a mechanical obstruction impedes venous inflow and/or cardiac output, such as with cardiac tamponade, tension pneumothorax, and massive pulmonary embolism (PE).

Some clinical presentations of shock and hypotension are readily categorized based on the history and physical exam. An elderly patient presenting with cough, tachypnea, fever, hypoxia, and hypotension can tentatively be diagnosed with distributive/septic shock due to pneumonia even prior to confirmatory testing, and the

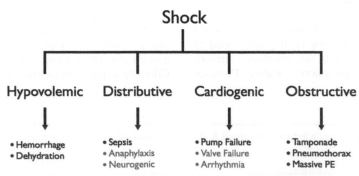

Fig. 1. Categories of shock. Categories of shock most amenable to diagnosis by bedside ultrasound are highlighted in dark font.

managing clinician often will initiate therapy before obtaining proof of the diagnosis. On the other hand, it may be difficult to differentiate profound hypovolemic shock due to a ruptured AAA from distributive shock in a patient with advanced urosepsis. Patients may not always exhibit classic clinical presentations, and signs and symptoms can be misleading. In addition, patients may have overlapping etiologies contributing to their shock state, such as distributive/septic shock that complicates a baseline severe cardiomyopathy. It is in these cases of undifferentiated shock that a bedside ultrasound evaluation of the underlying physiology and for exclusion of life-threatening diagnoses may prove most vital.

ULTRASOUND EVALUATION OF THE PATIENT IN SHOCK

A structured ultrasound protocol evaluating the heart, IVC, abdomen, aorta, and lungs can provide valuable information guiding the clinician to better differentiate between the etiologies of shock outlined above. Analogous to the FAST exam in trauma, such an ultrasound protocol serves as a standardized approach that may be committed to memory and easily followed in high-stress situations. It provides a systematic mental framework that facilitates the categorization of shock in the hypotensive patient, and in some cases may reveal the specific underlying cause of the patient's present illness. It also allows the clinician to make more informed decisions about initial fluid resuscitation and subsequent management of volume status. However, in contrast to the FAST exam, ultrasound evaluation of the critically ill medical patient is both technically and intellectually more challenging, reflecting the complexity of sick medical patients and the extensive differential diagnosis that must be considered. The FAST exam seeks to identify free fluid in key bodily compartments as an indication of traumatic sources of hemorrhage as well as cardiac tamponade. Ultrasound in critically ill patients incorporates a similar assessment but expands significantly on the techniques used and the target organs evaluated.

Ultrasound findings in any given disease state fall along a continuum of severity, which corresponds to the severity of the patient's underlying disease. Given the advanced stage of illness and extremes of physiology in critically ill patients in shock, ultrasound findings are less likely to be subtle in appearance and often more readily apparent and recognizable to the clinician sonographer. For example, the patient in extremis due to suspected massive PE may be too unstable to leave the resuscitation area to obtain CT confirmation of the diagnosis or await portable consultative echocardiography prior to key therapeutic interventions. Identification of gross RV dilation during a bedside ultrasound evaluation, combined with significant pretest clinical suspicion, may serve as strong enough evidence to warrant initiation of thrombolysis in certain cases.[19,20] On the other hand, in stable patients, a comprehensive echocardiographic exam may instead be obtained to more precisely grade the degree of RV dysfunction, a useful prognostic factor in the workup of PE. While consultative imaging will always have a role in providing comprehensive evaluations and for differentiating subtleties of disease, point-of-care ultrasound in the critically ill patient seeks to identify extremes in pathophysiology to better manage urgent patient care.

OVERVIEW OF ULTRASOUND PROTOCOLS

An ultrasound algorithm to evaluate critically ill patients with undifferentiated hypotension was first proposed by Rose and colleagues[21] in 2001, termed the UHP (Undifferentiated Hypotensive Patient) Ultrasound Protocol. The protocol incorporated 3 previously validated point-of-care ultrasound applications to identify reversible causes of hypotension. Relatively simple in scope, it consisted of a hepatorenal (Morison's pouch) view to evaluate for hemoperitoneum, a subxiphoid cardiac view to identify pericardial effusion, and a transverse sweep of the aorta to exclude AAA. In 2004, Jones and colleagues[22] expanded on this ultrasound protocol, naming it goal-directed ultrasound. The new protocol included additional abdominal (sagittal and transverse pelvis) and cardiac (parasternal long axis, apical 4-chamber) views, as well as an evaluation of the IVC to estimate volume status. Goal-directed ultrasound used immediately on patient arrival was compared with standard care for 15 minutes prior to goal-directed ultrasound. Immediate goal-directed ultrasound resulted in a narrowed differential diagnosis earlier in patient care, and the preliminary diagnosis turned out to be correct more frequently.

Since then, other protocols and different terminology have been proposed for an algorithmic ultrasound assessment of the patient in shock. The FATE (Focus Assessed Transthoracic Echocardiogram) protocol, performed by noncardiologists in the ICU setting, was proposed as an assessment of key determinants of hemodynamics in the critically ill.[23] The CAUSE exam (Cardiac Arrest Ultra-Sound Exam) highlighted the utility of ultrasound to rapidly identify reversible causes of non-arrhythmogenic cardiac arrest:

severe hypovolemia (such as from a ruptured AAA), cardiac tamponade, tension pneumothorax, and massive PE.[24] Along similar lines, the FEEL (Focused Echocardiography Evaluation in Life Support) protocol has been proposed as a rapid, point-of-care echocardiography protocol to be used in guiding peri-resuscitation care.[25,26] The ACES (Abdominal and Cardiac Evaluation with Sonography in Shock) protocol demonstrated how an integration of individual ultrasound findings facilitates categorization of the patient's underlying physiologic state of shock.[27]

Recently, more extensive protocols have been proposed under the title of the RUSH (Rapid Ultrasound in Shock and Hypotension) exam. Perera and colleagues[28] described a thorough ultrasound evaluation separated into 3 categories: the pump (focused echocardiogram for pericardial effusion, global LV contractility, and RV:LV ratio as a surrogate marker for massive PE), the tank (IVC for volume status, peritoneal and pleural cavities for free fluid), and the pipes (thoracic aorta for evidence of dissection, abdominal aorta for AAA, and the lower extremity veins for deep venous thrombosis). In their description of the RUSH exam, Weingart and colleagues[29] proposed the HI-MAP mnemonic to facilitate easy remembrance of the sequence of ultrasound evaluations, corresponding to the heart, IVC, Morison's pouch (representing an abdominal exam to identify free fluid), aorta, and pulmonary (**Fig. 2**). HI-MAP serves as a helpful tool to quickly recall the essential ultrasound applications in critically ill patients in shock or extremis.[8]

The proposed ultrasound algorithms need not be rigidly applied to completion in all patients. While a heart and IVC evaluation are typically of value in all critically ill patients presenting in shock, whether or not to perform the remaining components should be based on the specifics of the patient demographic and clinical presentation. For example, hypotension in an elderly patient with low back or flank pain suggests the possibility of ruptured AAA, and it is imperative that an ultrasound of the abdominal aorta be performed to assess for the presence or absence of this diagnosis. In comparison, hypotension in a young female patient with low back or pelvic pain raises the possibility of ruptured ectopic pregnancy, and an ultrasound of the abdomen and pelvis for identification of free fluid, in conjunction with a dipstick urine pregnancy test, is essential in this patient.

Similarly, interpretation of ultrasound findings can be made only within the clinical context of the patient's medical history and current presentation. To illustrate, the hypotensive young female patient with low back or pelvic pain and abdominal

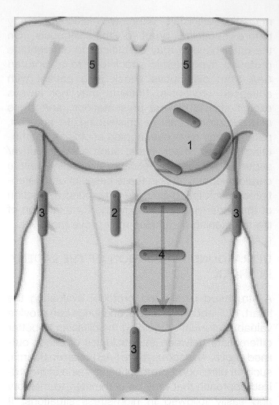

Fig. 2. RUSH protocol. 1, heart; 2, IVC; 3, abdomen; 4, aorta; 5, pulmonary.

free fluid on ultrasound suggests the diagnosis of ruptured ectopic pregnancy, which is all but confirmed if the dipstick urine pregnancy test is positive. On the contrary, the presence of peritoneal free fluid in a hypotensive patient of any age with pre-existing advanced cirrhosis may be an incidental finding and should not be relied on as the etiology of shock in this patient. In such a way, these protocols provide a mental framework for how point-of-care ultrasound may be applied to the critically ill patient, but at the same time must be adapted (both in terms of the specific components performed and how the results are interpreted) depending on the patient being cared for.

LIMITATIONS TO POINT-OF-CARE ULTRASOUND

The intent of clinician-performed ultrasound is not to replace consultative imaging. Instead, it is meant to be used for focused applications that answer specific clinical questions from the patient bedside. While point-of-care ultrasound can be extremely helpful to patient care, the clinician sonographer must also be aware of its limitations. For example, evaluation for valvular dysfunction is outside the scope of most emergency physicians and intensivists,[14] except in those who have received additional specialized training. Clinician sonographers may perform a focused echocardiogram to assess normal versus depressed or severely depressed systolic function when evaluating for cardiogenic shock, but a cardiogenic etiology also may be caused by acute valvular disease. Definitive exclusion of this diagnosis requires a comprehensive echocardiogram performed and interpreted by consultants.

Limitations of point-of-care ultrasound are covered in each of the following sections detailing the individual components of the proposed ultrasound protocol. It is vital that clinician sonographers be aware of these limitations when making patient care decisions based on their ultrasound findings.

COMPONENTS OF THE ULTRASOUND PROTOCOL: CARDIAC

Ultrasound evaluation of the patient in shock begins with a focused echocardiogram. Point-of-care echocardiography is a critical first-line test that can expedite the diagnostic evaluation and resuscitation of patients from the bedside. Its value lies in the ability to provide clinicians with real-time anatomic and physiologic information and the fact that it can be repeated after interventions to assess clinical response. Compared with comprehensive echocardiography, bedside cardiac ultrasound in the critically ill patient is a focused assessment to determine whether a patient's shock is due to pump failure (cardiogenic shock), inadequate preload (hypovolemic or distributive shock), or some form of mechanical obstruction (obstructive shock). Both the ASE and ACEP endorse the following clinical applications for focused cardiac ultrasound (FOCUS): pericardial effusion, global cardiac function, relative chamber size, and volume status.[14] Ultrasound in the critically ill patient begins by assessing for each of these findings.

The heart is imaged from multiple different views, and the findings seen on 1 view should be confirmed or refuted with another. A 2-MHz to 5-MHz phased array probe is used for cardiac ultrasound, since the small profile more easily fits between the ribs when attempting to obtain acoustic windows of the heart. There are 4 basic cardiac views: parasternal long axis, parasternal short axis, apical 4-chamber, and subcostal. If possible, the patient should be rolled into the left lateral decubitus position because this brings the heart closer to the anterior chest wall and improves imaging. The parasternal view is obtained by placing the probe to the left of the sternum and gently dragging it over the chest wall between the second and fifth intercostal spaces to obtain the best possible image. Once the parasternal long axis view is obtained, the probe can then be rotated 90° to obtain the parasternal short axis view. The apical 4-chamber view is obtained by placing the probe inferior to the left nipple in men or under the left breast in women and angling the face of the transducer up toward the base of the heart. The subcostal view is obtained by placing the probe just below the xiphoid process, using the left lobe of the liver as an acoustic window and projecting the face of the transducer up from the abdomen toward the heart.

Global Cardiac Function

Determination of global LV function is fundamental to the ultrasound evaluation of critically ill patients and has been shown to be predictive of clinical outcomes for a variety of disease states.[30–33] Assessment of systolic function is derived from qualitative evaluation of endocardial border excursion and myocardial thickening as seen from multiple views. Classification of LV function can be simplified into the following categories: severely depressed (ejection fraction [EF] <30%), moderately depressed (EF 30%–55%), and normal (EF >55%).[13,34,35] EFs in excess of 70% are considered hyperdynamic, which may appear as near obliteration of the ventricular cavity during systole. In critically ill patients, hyperdynamic EF usually reflects an underfilled LV, which may result from profound hypovolemia or an obstructive process (classically massive PE), or severe peripheral vasodilation, as occurs in distributive/septic shock. In nontrauma patients with undifferentiated symptomatic hypotension, an EF greater than 55% has been shown to be predictive of septic shock.[34]

While many quantitative measures of LV function exist (using M-mode, two-dimensional, or Doppler imaging), they may be limited by assumptions regarding LV shape, presence of extensive wall motion abnormalities, or sonographer skill. In the end, assessment of LV function is usually performed subjectively, with visual estimates by trained observers being similar or equal to calculations obtained by quantitative measures.[36–38] With focused education and training, emergency providers have demonstrated the ability to differentiate between normal and depressed LV systolic function (**Fig. 3**). Studies show that emergency providers can be trained to accurately determine LV function in hypotensive patients.[13] While noncardiologists tend to have more trouble categorizing patients with moderately depressed EFs,[13,35] clinician-performed echocardiography can effectively differentiate normal versus severely

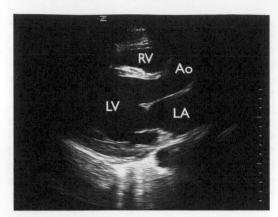

Fig. 3. Dilated cardiomyopathy. Parasternal long axis view of the heart showing a dilated LV as a result of chronically depressed EF. Ao, aortic root; LA, left atrium; LV, left ventricle; RV, right ventricle.

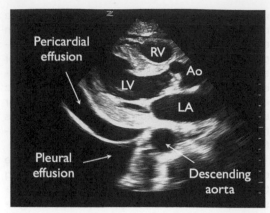

Fig. 4. Pericardial versus pleural effusion. Parasternal long axis view of the heart showing both a pericardial and pleural effusion.

depressed LV function. Accordingly, the intent of bedside echocardiography is not to distinguish more subtle differences in EF, but to identify extremes of LV dysfunction to appropriately categorize a critically ill patient's underlying state of shock.

Pericardial Effusions

Pericardial effusions are not an uncommon diagnosis in patients presenting with dyspnea or hypotension.[39,40] Patients with underlying pericardial effusions can have nonspecific symptoms such as cough, dyspnea on exertion, and fatigue, and physical exam findings may be equally nonspecific.[41–43] Studies have shown that bedside echocardiography performed by clinicians can detect the presence of pericardial effusions and positively impact patient management.[44–47] Pericardial effusions are defined by the presence of fluid (typically anechoic in appearance) between the epicardium and pericardium. They are caused by a variety of disorders (infection, malignancy, connective tissue disease, renal failure, trauma) and may also develop after cardiac surgery and invasive cardiac procedures (pacemaker placement, cardiac catheterization). Both their size and rate of accumulation are determining factors in terms of clinical and hemodynamic impact. Several studies have demonstrated that emergency physician-performed echocardiography has sensitivities approaching 100% for the detection of pericardial fluid.[2,12,40,48] While large pleural effusions may be misinterpreted as pericardial effusions, the descending thoracic aorta can be used to differentiate the 2 diagnoses. Pleural effusions run posterior or lateral to the descending thoracic aorta, whereas pericardial effusions track anteriorly or medially (**Fig. 4**).

Implicit in identifying effusions in critically ill patients in shock is the question of cardiac tamponade. While many would argue that cardiac tamponade is largely a clinical diagnosis, echocardiography can reveal findings suggestive of pre-tamponade or early tamponade states.[49] The hallmark echocardiographic finding in cardiac tamponade is RV free-wall inversion during ventricular diastole.[50] Additional findings include RA inversion during ventricular systole (most common and earliest finding), increased respiratory variation of Doppler inflow velocities (echocardiographic equivalent of pulsus paradoxus), and a dilated IVC with diminished respirophasic variation.[51,52] In trauma patients, bedside echocardiography has been shown to result in earlier diagnosis of cardiac tamponade and decreased time to the operating room or thoracotomy.[2,48,53] This time-saving value of bedside ultrasound can be extrapolated to its use in the identification and management of pericardial effusions in critically ill medical patients. In addition, for patients with hemodynamic compromise prompting emergent pericardial effusion drainage, ultrasound can be used to determine the best approach for pericardiocentesis and then guide its performance. Ultrasound-guided pericardiocentesis has been shown to increase success rates and to decrease the risk of complications, such as myocardial puncture, coronary vascular injury, pneumothorax, abdominal visceral puncture, and diaphragmatic injury.[54–58]

Right Ventricular Enlargement

The ability to assess for right heart failure may prove vital in the assessment of patients with undifferentiated shock. Patients with right heart dysfunction are treated differently from those with left heart failure, and their management can be quite challenging. Hypotensive patients with right heart failure may worsen with aggressive fluid resuscitation[59,60]; instead, treatment or reversal of the etiology of the RV fluid or pressure overload is key. While RV systolic function can be qualitatively evaluated in a manner similar to that of the LV (by assessing endocardial border excursion and myocardial thickening), right ventricular enlargement is often used as a surrogate for dysfunction. The normal RV is thin walled and sensitive to changes in load; consequently, small changes in pressure result in large changes in ventricular volume. RV enlargement is the physiologic response to RV pressure or volume overload.[61] The normal ratio between RV and LV sizes (measured at the tips of the atrioventricular valves on the apical 4-chamber view) is 0.6. When the RV is equal in size to the LV, RV dilation is graded as moderate; when the RV is larger than the LV, RV dilation is graded as severe.[62]

Just as the question of cardiac tamponade is implicit in identifying pericardial effusions, so is the question of PE when assessing for right ventricular enlargement. While the appropriate clinical setting may suggest the diagnosis of PE, echocardiography alone (even when comprehensive) is not entirely accurate in establishing the diagnosis.[63–65] Other causes of right ventricular enlargement must be considered, including RV infarction, pulmonary hypertension, and chronic obstructive pulmonary disease. In addition to RV enlargement, echocardiography in patients with massive PE may also demonstrate a hyperdynamic and underfilled LV (**Fig. 5**). The LV, which normally has a circular appearance on the parasternal short axis view, can appear D-shaped due to flattening of the interventricular septum as a result of increased RV pressures. In some instances, echocardiography may reveal embolized venous thrombus in the RA in transit to the pulmonary circulation. Although infrequent, with reported incidences ranging from 3% to 18% in acute PE, venous thromboembolism in transit may be considered direct evidence of PE.[66–68] McConnell's sign, a distinct regional pattern of RV dysfunction with akinesia of the mid-free wall but normal motion at the apex, was originally found to have a specificity of 94% for the diagnosis of acute PE.[69] However, subsequent studies have not validated this finding, and some suggest that RV apical contractility is not spared and McConnell's sign is more of a visual illusion due to tethering of the RV apex to the LV.[70]

INFERIOR VENA CAVA

Determination of intravascular volume status can be difficult in the critically ill patient in shock. A patient with septic shock and hypotension may still be intravascularly volume depleted despite having received multiple liters of intravenous fluids within the initial few hours of presentation. The patient may benefit from additional volume loading, and initiation of vasopressors prematurely to augment blood pressure may have adverse consequences on perfusion of vital organs. In addition, a patient with pre-existing cardiomyopathy may present volume depleted in septic shock. Volume management in such patients is tenuous, since excessive fluid infusion may quickly lead to volume overload and flash pulmonary edema. As a capacitance vessel, the IVC can accommodate varying amounts of blood, and its size fluctuates depending on a patient's intravascular volume. Accordingly, ultrasound measurements of the IVC can be used as a sonographic estimate of intravascular volume status.

The IVC is imaged from the anterior abdomen in a longitudinal orientation using a subcostal sagittal approach,[17,18] positioning the probe slightly to the right of midline. A 2-MHz to 5-MHz curvilinear probe is frequently used for this exam, although a microconvex or phased array probe can also be used. The IVC is assessed for both vessel diameter and respirophasic changes. IVC diameter is measured from inner wall to inner wall in the anterior-posterior dimension, either just caudal to the confluence of the IVC with the hepatic veins or 2 to 3 cm caudal to the atriocaval junction (**Fig. 6**).[71] IVC diameter is dynamic and changes size depending on the phase of the patient's respiratory cycle. In a spontaneously breathing patient, negative thoracic pressure is generated during inspiration, which draws blood from the extrathoracic

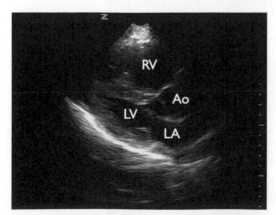

Fig. 5. Right ventricular enlargement. Parasternal long axis view of the heart showing severe right ventricular enlargement and a small, underfilled LV.

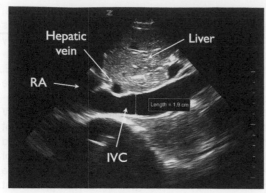

Fig. 6. IVC. Subcostal long axis view of the IVC with diameter measurement.

vena cava into the chest. As a result, IVC diameter is greatest during expiration (IVC$_e$) and exhibits varying degrees of collapse during inspiration (IVC$_i$). Testing for IVC collapse can be augmented by asking the patient to sniff, or inspire forcefully (the so-called sniff test), when able to follow commands. The percentage collapse of IVC diameter during inspiration has been termed the caval index (also collapsibility index): (IVC$_e$ − IVC$_i$) / IVC$_e$. Visualization of relative IVC size throughout the respiratory cycle may be facilitated using M-mode ultrasound (**Fig. 7**).

Many studies have investigated how IVC diameter and the caval index relate to intravascular volume, often estimated by central venous pressure (CVP) measurements, a commonly used although imperfect measure of volume status.[72–74] Absolute IVC diameter has been shown to

decrease in size in response to decreasing intravascular volume[75–78] and may be used to follow relative volume status, similar to trending CVP measurements. However, significant variation in baseline IVC diameter from individual to individual limits the value of isolated IVC diameter measurements.[17,79,80] In comparison, respiratory variation in IVC size has better predictive value for estimation of right-sided filling pressures than static measurements of IVC diameter. Greater than 50% IVC collapse with inspiration (caval index >0.5) predicts CVP less than 10 mm Hg; conversely, less than 50% IVC collapse (caval index <0.5) predicts CVP greater than 10 mm Hg.[17,18,81]

Tables correlating IVC measurements with distinct CVP ranges (0–5, 5–10, 10–15, and 15–20 mm Hg) are commonly included in textbooks on the subject,[82,83] although the data supporting such a precise relationship is minimal.[84] While individual IVC diameters and caval indices may not accurately correspond to specific numerical CVP values, they may better predict patients at the extremes of volume depletion or volume overload (**Table 1**).[18] A small (<1.5 cm) IVC$_e$ that shows complete (or near complete) collapse with inspiration indicates that the hypotensive patient in shock is volume depleted (**Fig. 8**). Such patients likely will benefit from aggressive volume loading. A large (>2.5 cm) IVC$_e$ that shows no (or minimal) change with inspiration, referred to as a plethoric IVC,[18,85] can be seen in patients who are volume overloaded (**Fig. 9**). However, a plethoric IVC may be observed in a number of other conditions (described further below) and does not necessarily reflect a state of intravascular volume overload.

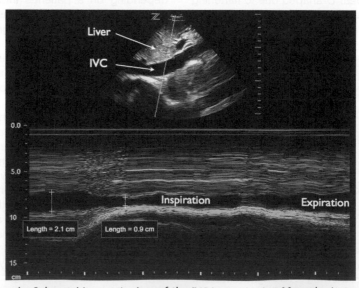

Fig. 7. IVC with M-mode. Subcostal long axis view of the IVC imaged using M-mode during inspiration.

Table 1
IVC measurement findings at the extremes of volume depletion and volume overload

Volume Status	Diameter (cm)	Inspiration	CVP (mm Hg)
Volume depletion	<1.5	Complete collapse	<5
Volume overload (possible)	>2.5	No collapse	>20

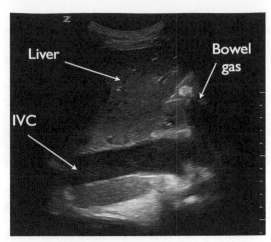

Fig. 9. Plethoric IVC. Subcostal long axis view of the IVC showing a dilated diameter in volume overload.

While a collapsed IVC suggests that volume resuscitation is warranted, a plethoric IVC as an isolated finding should not be relied on to discontinue further volume infusion.

Increased right atrial pressures (and consequently increased CVPs) are present in isolated right-sided heart failure and chronic pulmonary hypertension.[86,87] In these patients, a plethoric IVC can be seen, although left-sided filling pressures may be suboptimal despite elevated right-sided pressures. Ultrasound evaluation of the IVC for determination of effective intravascular volume is of less utility in these clinical settings, and a plethoric IVC does not exclude the possibility that further volume loading will augment cardiac output.

A plethoric IVC may be a clue to cardiogenic and obstructive etiologies of shock. RV failure and/or total body volume overload often accompanies LV failure in chronic cardiomyopathies. Blood flow backs up from the right heart and fills the IVC as a capacitance vessel, resulting in a plethoric IVC. A plethoric IVC is also observed in acute obstructive processes that impede venous inflow into the heart, such as cardiac tamponade, tension pneumothorax, and massive PE. In these cases, a plethoric IVC reflects impaired filling of the heart and not intravascular volume overload. In fact, patients with obstructive shock due to cardiac tamponade and tension pneumothorax benefit from aggressive volume infusion until more definitive therapies to relieve the obstruction (ie, pericardiocentesis and chest needle decompression) can be performed. Care must be taken with fluid resuscitation in patients with massive PE, since overaggressive volume infusion may increase RV wall stress and induce worsening ischemia.[59,60]

When patients are mechanically ventilated with positive pressure ventilation, respirophasic changes in IVC diameter are reversed. Since positive pressures are generated during inspiration, blood is forced from the chest into the extrathoracic vena cava, and the IVC slightly distends as a result. An underfilled IVC is more compliant and increases in size more during inspiration than a relatively well-filled IVC. The percentage distention of IVC diameter during inspiration in patients receiving positive pressure ventilation has been termed the distensibility index: (IVC_i − IVC_e) / IVC_e. The distensibility index has been well studied in the ICU,[88,89] where patients frequently require mechanical ventilation. A threshold value of 18% dichotomizes those patients who increase their cardiac output in response to further volume infusion from those who do not. While 18% does represent a discrete cutoff, patients are more likely to exhibit or lack fluid responsiveness the further the distensibility index separates from this threshold value.[88]

ABDOMEN

The FAST exam is perhaps the hallmark clinician-performed ultrasound application. From the early

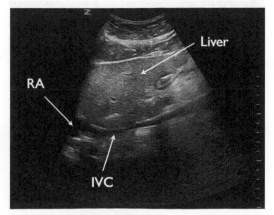

Fig. 8. Collapsed IVC. Subcostal long axis view of the IVC showing near complete collapse during inspiration in volume depletion.

1970s onward, the utility of ultrasound for detecting hemoperitoneum and resuscitating trauma patients has been thoroughly investigated.[90–94] The FAST exam has been shown to decrease the time to recognition of abdominal trauma and operative intervention as well as to decrease hospital costs and resource use.[3,95,96] In recognition of these benefits, the FAST exam is now included in the ATLS protocol of the American College of Sugeons[8] and in the Eastern Association for the Surgery of Trauma (EAST) guidelines for the management of blunt abdominal trauma.[97] Likewise, the American College of Radiology recommends the use of ultrasound to evaluate for free or localized intra-abdominal fluid collections.[98]

While originally applied to trauma patients, use of the FAST exam has expanded in scope to include critically ill medical patients as well. Perhaps the best example of the use of the FAST exam in non-trauma patients is for the diagnosis of hemoperitoneum in patients with suspected ectopic pregnancy. The presence of intraperitoneal fluid in pregnant patients without a definite intrauterine pregnancy is indirect evidence but highly suggestive for an ectopic pregnancy and can be life saving.[99] Interrogation of the hepatorenal space (Morison's pouch) in the right upper quadrant (RUQ) is considered standard practice in the ultrasound evaluation of the first-trimester pregnancy patient with abdominal pain or vaginal bleeding. Hemoperitoneum secondary to a variety of emergent causes, such as arterial aneurysm rupture, splenic rupture, or iatrogenic injury, can likewise be detected with the FAST exam.

The FAST exam consists of 4 standard views (RUQ, left upper quadrant [LUQ], pelvis, and subcostal cardiac) for the identification of fluid in the peritoneal cavity and within the pericardial sac. A 2-MHz to 5-MHz curvilinear probe is typically used for this exam, although a microconvex or phased array probe may also suffice. While ultrasound can detect as little as 100 mL of free fluid in the peritoneal cavity,[82,91,100] fluid collections in the range of 250 to 500 mL (which indicates hemodynamically significant bleeding when due to hemoperitoneum) or greater are more reliably detected during the FAST exam.[101–103] The location of accumulating fluid is dependent on patient positioning as well as the source of bleeding. In recent years, research has demonstrated the value of including views of the thorax to assess for hemothorax and pneumothorax.[104–106] This extended version of the FAST exam is referred to as the E-FAST and includes views of both hemithoraces at the level of the diaphragm-abdominal interface as well as over the anterior chest wall (see pulmonary section).

The RUQ view is obtained by placing the probe in the coronal plane. The liver serves as the acoustic window and, given its size, the RUQ view can be imaged from the anterior axillary, mid-axillary, or posterior axillary line (**Fig. 10**). The RUQ view includes the interrogation of 3 distinct areas: the subdiaphragmatic space, Morison's pouch, and the inferior pole of the right kidney. Morison's pouch is a potential, dependent space between the liver and right kidney and, in the supine patient, is the most sensitive location for the detection of free fluid in the upper abdomen. To interrogate the right subdiaphragmatic space and the inferior pole of the right kidney, the probe is repositioned cephalad and caudad, respectively.

The LUQ view is likewise obtained by placing the probe in the coronal plane. Since the spleen is more limited in size and more posterior in location, the LUQ view is best imaged from the posterior axillary line. The LUQ view similarly interrogates 3 distinct areas: the subdiaphragmatic space, the splenorenal space, and the inferior pole of the left kidney. While the splenorenal space is often equated to Morison's pouch, the phrenocolic ligament closely apposes the spleen and kidney, thus limiting the flow of intraperitoneal fluid into this area. Consequently, considerable amounts of free intraperitoneal fluid may accumulate in the subdiaphragmatic space or at the inferior pole of the left kidney before any can be visualized in the splenorenal space (**Fig. 11**). To interrogate the left subdiaphragmatic space and the inferior pole of the left kidney, the probe is repositioned cephalad and caudad, respectively.

The pelvis view is obtained by placing the probe just above the pubic symphysis, using the urinary bladder as an acoustic window. Since the pelvis is a ring-like structure, the probe must be angled

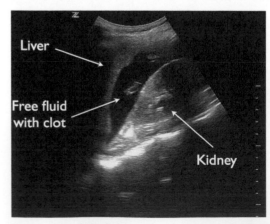

Fig. 10. RUQ free fluid. Coronal view of the RUQ showing free fluid and echogenic clot in Morison's pouch.

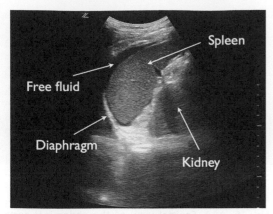

Fig. 11. LUQ free fluid. Coronal view of the LUQ showing free fluid surrounding the spleen.

caudally, deep into the pelvis, to visualize relevant structures. The pelvis view interrogates the rectovesicular space in men and the rectouterine space (pouch of Douglas) in women. The sagittal view of the pelvis is obtained by placing the probe in the midline sagittal plane. Once a sagittal view has been obtained, the probe can then be rotated 90° to obtain a transverse view of the pelvis. Compared with the transverse view, the sagittal view may be more sensitive for detecting small amounts of pelvic fluid (**Fig. 12**). Difficulty obtaining a pelvis view may be secondary to a decompressed bladder or a probe position that is too cephalad.

The subcostal view of the heart is obtained by placing the probe just below the xiphoid process. This view uses the left lobe of the liver as an acoustic window and requires that the face of the transducer be angled up from the abdomen toward the heart. Difficulty obtaining a subcostal view may be secondary to probe positioning that is too caudad or insufficient depth leaving key

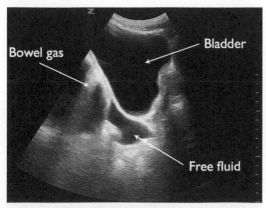

Fig. 12. Pelvic free fluid. Sagittal view of the pelvis showing free fluid in the rectovesicular space adjacent to bowel gas and a full bladder.

structures out of view. If the subcostal view is limited, an alternative window, such as a parasternal or apical view, should be used.

AORTA

Acute aortic disease should always be considered in critically ill patients presenting with undifferentiated shock. While aortic emergencies such as aneurysms and dissection may present classically with abdominal or flank pain or chest pain radiating to the back, they may also present in a more nonspecific manner with syncope, dizziness, neurologic findings, end-organ ischemia, or cardiac arrest. Aortic disease is often not detected on physical exam[107,108] and patients may remain asymptomatic until rupture or dissection occurs. Prompt intervention is key, and, in these patients, bedside ultrasound of the aorta may expedite care and be life saving.[109,110]

For AAA, clinician-performed ultrasound is an excellent noninvasive screening modality, with sensitivities ranging between 94% and 98%.[11,111–113] The ability to detect AAA can improve patient outcomes, as mortality has been shown to decrease if the diagnosis is made prior to or shortly after rupture.[114–116] While ultrasound is an excellent tool for detecting the presence of AAA, it is limited in terms of the ability to assess for rupture. In rare instances (<4% of cases), ultrasound may demonstrate findings consistent with rupture: usually retroperitoneal hematoma, although thrombus interruption, aortic wall interruption, or free intraperitoneal fluid can also be seen.

In aortic dissection, mortality likewise can be high, and, when involving the ascending aorta, early surgical intervention is known to improve patient outcomes. While suboptimal in terms of sensitivity, bedside ultrasound can have important clinical impact, as visualization of an intimal flap may influence further diagnostic evaluation and expedite clinical management (**Fig. 13**). Transthoracic echocardiography has sensitivities reported between 59% and 83% and specificities between 63% and 93% for the diagnosis of aortic dissection.[117–119] Its sensitivity in identifying ascending aortic dissections (where the diagnosis needs to be made more rapidly) is higher compared with descending thoracic aortic dissections.[119] For patients in whom a dissection flap is visualized, bedside ultrasound can identify those features of ascending dissection that indicate high risk and impending rupture: severe proximal aorta dilation, pericardial effusion, and aortic insufficiency.[120]

The abdominal aorta is imaged in both the transverse and sagittal planes. A 2-MHz to 5-MHz

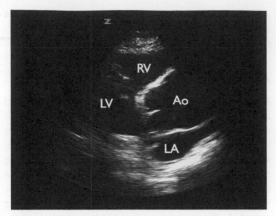

Fig. 13. Dilated aortic root. Parasternal long axis view of the heart showing a severely dilated aortic root. A mobile dissection flap was visualized on real-time imaging.

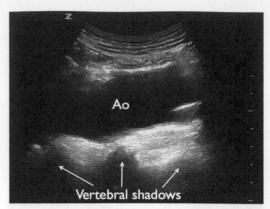

Fig. 15. AAA. Sagittal view of the abdominal aorta showing an aneurysm.

curvilinear probe is typically used for this exam, although a microconvex or phased array probe may also suffice. Imaging begins in the subxiphoid area, using the vertebral body of the spine as a landmark to identify the aorta. The aorta is located anterior to the vertebral body and toward the patient's left (**Fig. 14**). The proximal, mid-, and distal abdominal aortic diameters are measured from outer wall to outer wall in the anterior-posterior dimension using images obtained in the transverse plane. Below the aortic bifurcation, the iliac arteries should likewise be measured. Performing measurements in the transverse (as opposed to the sagittal) plane decreases the chance of obtaining off-axis views and consequently underestimating aortic size. Once the abdominal aorta has been imaged from proximal to distal levels, the probe is then rotated 90° into the sagittal plane (**Fig. 15**). The sagittal view allows for easier visualization of focal

outpouchings (ie, saccular aneurysms) and better localization of any noted abnormalities along the long axis of the body. When imaging is limited by overlying bowel gas, graded compression can improve the view; however, technically limited studies may still occur in 5% to 10% of ultrasound scans.[121,122]

The thoracic aorta can be imaged through a combination of multiple different views. The aortic root can be interrogated and measured on the parasternal long axis cardiac view. The suprasternal view, obtained with the transducer placed in the suprasternal notch, can be used to evaluate the aortic arch. Portions of the descending thoracic aorta can be visualized in the far field of both the parasternal and apical cardiac views. Abdominal views of the aorta may also be used to determine if an abnormality extends down to the abdominal aorta (**Fig. 16**). If an intimal flap is thought to be seen, it is important to confirm or refute this finding with a second view. In addition, echocardiography can be used to assess for high-

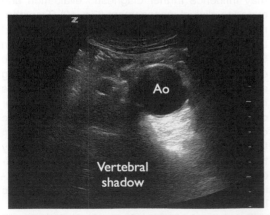

Fig. 14. AAA. Transverse view of the abdominal aorta showing an aneurysm.

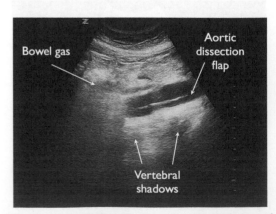

Fig. 16. Abdominal aortic dissection. Sagittal view of the abdominal aorta showing a dissection flap.

risk features of aortic dissection such as pericardial effusion and aortic insufficiency.

PULMONARY

Traditionally, many believed that ultrasound had little utility in the assessment of the lungs.[123,124] Since ultrasound waves are strongly scattered by air, it was thought that sonography was not a useful modality for imaging the lungs or evaluating for associated pathology. However, pulmonary ultrasound has proved to be a valuable aid in the diagnosis of a variety of pathologic conditions, including pneumothorax, pulmonary edema, pleural effusion, and alveolar consolidation.[15,16,125]

Pneumothorax

Pulmonary ultrasound has been extensively studied in the diagnosis of pneumothorax in trauma patients and has demonstrated sensitivity superior to that of chest radiography.[126–128] Pneumothorax is not an uncommon phenomenon in critically ill patients with medical disease. Pneumothorax may occur as a complication of obstructive lung disease, as in severe asthma and exacerbations of chronic obstructive pulmonary disease, or due to excessive alveolar pressures generated in patients receiving mechanical positive pressure ventilation. Pneumothorax may also occur iatrogenically following invasive procedures, such as insertion of internal jugular or subclavian vein catheters, cardiac pacemaker placement, or pericardiocentesis.

Assessment for pneumothorax is performed from the anterior thorax in a sagittal orientation in the midclavicular line. A 5-MHz to 10-MHz linear array probe is preferred due to of better visualization of the superficial structures imaged during this exam, although a microconvex or curvilinear probe set to shallow depths may also suffice. Typically the second to fifth intercostal spaces are evaluated, although more extensive evaluation of the chest wall has been proposed for certain purposes, such as identification of the lung point and for estimation of pneumothorax size (described further later).[125,127,129] A more comprehensive assessment of the chest also may be indicated when loculated pneumothorax is suspected.[125,127]

Presence or absence of pneumothorax is determined through an evaluation of the pleural interface. Whereas ultrasound waves are scattered once they reach the air-filled alveoli, sonography is able to visualize the pleural surface. In the absence of pneumothorax, movement of the parietal and visceral pleura against one another results in a shimmering or glistening appearance termed lung sliding.[15,16,125] Lung sliding is a dynamic finding seen only on real-time imaging, although M-mode ultrasound may be used to document lung sliding on still images. Lack of chest wall tissue movement appears as repeating horizontal lines in the near field, whereas sliding of the visceral and parietal pleura results in a granular appearance in the far field. Together, the appearance of the M-mode image has been likened to waves on a beach and termed the seashore sign (**Fig. 17**).[15,16,125] In

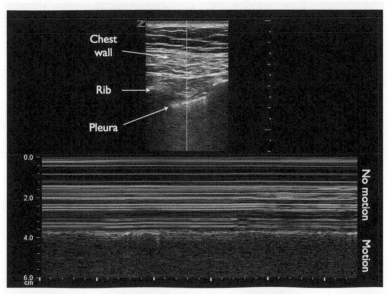

Fig. 17. Normal lung with M-mode. Sagittal view of the chest at the pleural interface imaged using M-mode shows the appearance of normal lung: the seashore sign.

the presence of a pneumothorax, air separates the parietal pleura from the visceral pleura, and lung sliding is absent on ultrasound. The pleural surface appears as a static linear stripe on real-time imaging, lacking its normal shimmering appearance. When imaged using M-mode, repeating horizontal lines are seen across the entire screen in both the near and far field, resulting in an image referred to as the bar code sign (**Fig. 18**).[101,125]

It has been proposed that the size of a pneumothorax may be estimated by performing a more thorough sonographic evaluation of the chest wall.[125,127,129] Moving from the most superior portion of the chest (where air from a small pneumothorax first collects) to more dependent regions (which are only affected by larger pneumothoraces) may be useful in mapping out the limits of a pneumothorax. The transition point between the presence and absence of lung sliding, corresponding to the limits of an incomplete pneumothorax along the chest wall, has been termed the lung point and is considered to be pathognomonic for pneumothorax.[127,129,130] The lung point is a dynamic finding where absent lung sliding alternates with the intermittent appearance of normal lung sliding, all while the ultrasound probe is held stationary at a particular location on the chest wall. This phenomenon is caused by transient contact of visceral against parietal pleura when inspiration increases lung volume and therefore increases lung surface area in contact with the chest wall.[129,130] Tension pneumothorax should result in the absence of lung sliding throughout the affected hemithorax, since accumulating air

completely separates underlying lung from the chest wall.

Absent lung sliding is not pathognomonic for pneumothorax and may be seen in other conditions. While pulmonary ultrasound has been shown to have excellent sensitivity for identifying the presence of pneumothorax, especially in trauma, the specificity of absent lung sliding for the diagnosis of pneumothorax is limited in medically complex patient populations.[15,127] Absence of lung sliding, mimicking pneumothorax, may also be seen with pleural blebs, adhesions, and scarring.[15,127,131] In addition, absence of lung sliding unilaterally over one hemithorax may be seen with right or left mainstem intubation.[132,133] A thorough evaluation of the chest wall demonstrating the presence of lung sliding safely rules out pneumothorax, especially tension pneumothorax as a cause of hypoxia or hypotension. However, other conditions need to be considered when lung sliding is absent, and additional confirmatory imaging may be necessary.

Pulmonary Edema

While ultrasonographic signs of pulmonary edema were first identified more than a decade ago,[134] only in recent years have they started to be incorporated into clinical practice in the ED and ICU. Pulmonary edema is a common reason for presentations to the hospital with acute shortness of breath. Cardiogenic shock results in severe pulmonary edema as poor cardiac output causes backup of fluid into the lungs. Early pulmonary

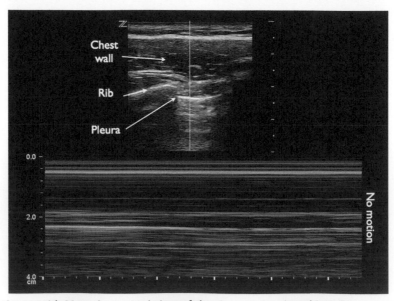

Fig. 18. Pneumothorax with M-mode. Sagittal view of the chest at the pleural interface imaged using M-mode shows the appearance of a pneumothorax: the bar code sign.

edema manifests as fluid accumulates in the lung interstitium, which can be detected using ultrasound as sonographic B-lines. As pulmonary edema becomes more severe, the alveoli begin to fill with fluid.

Comet tails are a type of reverberation artifact that originate from irregularities at the pleural surface and are visualized during ultrasound of normal lung. They appear as short, vertical echogenic lines that extend from the pleural interface and fade within several centimeters (**Fig. 19**).[101,125] Comet-tail artifacts move along with normal lung sliding and their presence excludes underlying pneumothorax at that position on the chest wall.[125,135] Sonographic B-lines are vertical echogenic lines that extend from the pleural surface all the way through the far field without fading (**Fig. 20**). It is important that imaging depth be set to 16 to 18 cm to differentiate comet-tail artifacts that fade within several centimeters from sonographic B-lines that extend all the way to the end of the screen. Pulmonary edema results in multiple (≥3) B-lines within a single intercostal space. The B-lines correspond to thickened interlobular septa as they swell with extravascular lung water.[136,137] B-lines appear diffusely across both hemithoraces in acute pulmonary edema, and this sonographic finding has been referred to as the interstitial syndrome (**Fig. 21**).[15,16,138] As pulmonary edema becomes more severe, individual B-lines may coalesce and the entire intercostal space appears hyperechoic, which has been referred to as white lung (**Fig. 22**).[139–141] Conversely, as pulmonary edema resolves with treatment, B-lines have been shown to disappear accordingly.[140,142]

Similar to evaluation for pneumothorax, evaluation for sonographic B-lines is performed from the anterior thorax in a sagittal orientation, typically in the second or third intercostal space in

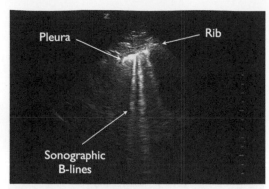

Fig. 20. Sonographic B-lines. Sagittal view of the chest at a single intercostal space showing sonographic B-lines.

the midclavicular line. The exam may be extended to the upper lateral chest wall to improve sensitivity.[143–145] However, in critically ill patients who are hypoxic due to severe pulmonary edema or hypotensive due to cardiogenic shock, views of the anterior chest only should be sufficient.[146] More dependent regions of the lung (posteriorly when the patient is supine or inferiorly with the patient upright) are more extensively perfused with blood, and scattered B-lines can be a normal finding there.[145,147] In distinction from the pulmonary scan for pneumothorax, in which a high frequency linear array probe is used to focus on superficial structures at the pleural interface, ultrasound evaluation for pulmonary edema should be performed with a lower-frequency curvilinear, microconvex, or phased array probe set to depths of 16 to 18 cm. A typical linear array probe images in the range of 3 to 6 cm, and both comet-tail artifacts and sonographic B-lines may extend through

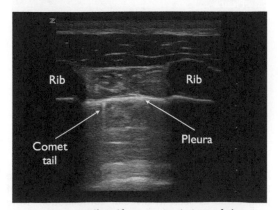

Fig. 19. Comet-tail artifact. Sagittal view of the chest at the pleural interface showing normal comet-tail artifact.

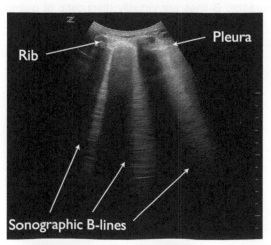

Fig. 21. Pulmonary edema. Sagittal view of the chest showing multiple sonographic B-lines in multiple intercostal spaces as seen in pulmonary edema.

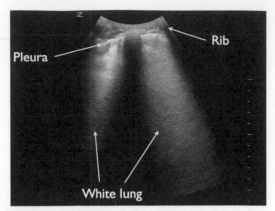

Fig. 22. Severe pulmonary edema. Sagittal view of the chest showing multiple hyperechoic intercostal spaces (white lung) as seen in severe pulmonary edema.

the far field at such shallow depths, potentially confusing the 2 findings.

Sonographic B-lines are not specific to pulmonary edema and may be seen in other processes that affect the interstitium, including interstitial pneumonias and chronic conditions such as pulmonary fibrosis.[148–150] Acute respiratory distress syndrome (ARDS), commonly encountered in the ICU, may also result in sonographic B-lines; however, the B-lines in ARDS are interspersed among areas of normal lung sliding, corresponding to the patchy airspace involvement in this condition (**Fig. 23**).[141] In addition, a thickened pleural line is often visualized in areas of the lung affected by ARDS.[141,151] When sonographic B-lines exhibit a bilateral and diffuse pattern, pulmonary edema is the most likely underlying process. Combined with echocardiographic findings of a low EF and plethoric IVC, especially when seen in the correct clinical context, sonographic B-lines are virtually diagnostic of pulmonary edema.

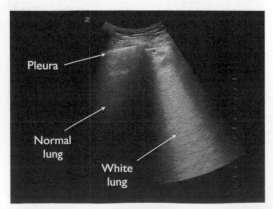

Fig. 23. ARDS. Sagittal view of the chest showing a hyperechoic intercostal space (white lung) adjacent to normal-appearing lung as seen in ARDS.

Alveolar Consolidation

Stemming from beliefs that ultrasound lacks utility in diagnosing lung pathology, it is not well appreciated that alveolar consolidation can be visualized with ultrasound. Although the identification of pneumothorax and pulmonary edema relies on interpretation of artifacts arising at the pleural surface, alveolar consolidation results in fluid-filled lung tissue that is well penetrated by ultrasound waves.[15,16,152] Consolidated lung has a tissue-like sonographic appearance similar to that of liver parenchyma, which has been termed hepatization of the lung (**Fig. 24**).[125,141,153] Distinct from the liver, alveolar consolidation frequently demonstrates sonographic air bronchograms, which appear as punctate or linear hyperechoic opacities within the consolidated lung tissue.[125,141,153] In addition, the interface between consolidated and aerated lung has a characteristic appearance. Tissue-like alveolar consolidation is bordered by an irregular, jagged hyperechoic line, representing scattering of ultrasound waves by aerated lung (see **Fig. 24**).[125,141,153] While alveolar consolidations do have a characteristic sonographic appearance, they may result from variable underlying causes, commonly infectious but also mechanical (bronchial obstruction), hydrostatic (pulmonary edema), and traumatic (pulmonary contusion). Sonographic visualization of alveolar consolidation may prove useful when searching for an underlying cause for hypoxia or an infectious source for septic shock, especially given the not infrequent poor quality of portable chest radiographs obtained in critically ill patients in respiratory distress.[154,155]

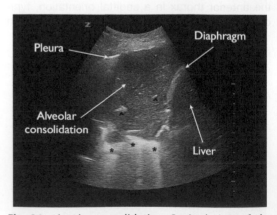

Fig. 24. Alveolar consolidation. Sagittal view of the RUQ above the diaphragm showing hepatization of lung tissue as seen in alveolar consolidation. Note the hyperechoic sonographic air bronchograms (^) and the interface between consolidated and aerated lung (*).

Pleural Effusion

Unlike the more novel applications of pulmonary ultrasound discussed above, use of ultrasound for the diagnosis of pleural effusion is well established.[124,156] It may be detected during a dedicated pulmonary ultrasound evaluation or as part of an abdominal exam (RUQ and LUQ sub-diaphragmatic views) or during echocardiography (parasternal long axis and apical views). Pleural effusions are common in critically ill medical patients and may result from cardiac failure, volume overload states, parapneumonic effusions, or empyema. Large pleural effusions can cause significant respiratory compromise and hypoxia. However, identification of a pleural effusion by it-self generally does not account for hypotension in critically ill medical patients in shock, as may be the case with detection of a large hemothorax in trauma patients.

INTEGRATION OF SONOGRAPHIC FINDINGS IN SHOCK

While individual ultrasound findings may be suggestive of certain shock states, integrating a combination of findings can more effectively narrow the differential by ruling out certain condi-tions and, in some cases, may definitively estab-lish the diagnosis. It is this integration of the entire ultrasound evaluation that makes protocols such as the RUSH exam particularly useful in correctly classifying a patient's underlying physio-logic state of shock (**Table 2**).

To illustrate, a depressed EF by itself does not necessarily establish the etiology of shock as solely cardiogenic, since patients may have pre-existing cardiomyopathy or have a depressed EF due to advanced sepsis. Depressed EF in conjunction with a plethoric IVC and diffuse, bilat-eral B-lines is much more compelling in establish-ing a diagnosis of cardiogenic shock. Conversely, a normal or hyperdynamic LV EF does not always eliminate the possibility of cardiogenic shock.

Acute valvular disease, such as acute aortic or mitral insufficiency, or right-sided myocardial infarction can also lead to cardiogenic shock. While it has already been stated that evaluation for valvular disease is outside the scope of most emergency physicians and intensivists, surrogate findings may still be helpful. A plethoric IVC should be present with significant right-sided myocardial infarctions, and diffuse, bilateral B-lines should be seen in acute aortic or mitral insufficiency.

In hypovolemic shock, ultrasound evaluation typically reveals a hyperdynamic EF, collapsed IVC, and absence of B-lines. LV dimensions may appear small due to diminished intravascular volume. Other findings from the ultrasound protocol may reveal the specific reason for the hypovolemia, such as a dilated aortic diameter in an elderly patient with a ruptured AAA or a large amount of peritoneal free fluid in a young female patient with a ruptured ectopic pregnancy.

In septic and other forms of distributive shock, again a hyperdynamic EF, collapsed IVC, and absence of B-lines are characteristic. In more advanced stages of septic shock, cardiac dys-function may occur and a depressed EF may be observed. A plethoric IVC may coexist with hypovolemic and septic shock in patients with chronic pulmonary hypertension or right-sided heart failure. While a collapsed IVC indicates intra-vascular volume depletion in the hypotensive patient, a plethoric IVC does not necessarily mean a patient is volume overloaded.

In obstructive shock, the IVC appears plethoric. When the cause of obstruction is cardiac tampo-nade, fluid is seen circumferentially surrounding the heart, and right atrial and/or ventricular inver-sion may be appreciated. With tension pneumo-thorax, lung sliding is absent over the affected chest, typically across the entire hemithorax. In the case of massive PE, a small, hyperdynamic LV, flattened interventricular septum, and severe RV enlargement are often observed. While not specifically described as part of the protocol detailed earlier, identification of a concomitant

Table 2
Common findings during the ultrasound evaluation of critically ill patients according to category of shock

	Hypovolemic	Distributive	Cardiogenic	Obstructive
Heart	Small, hyperdynamic	Hyperdynamic	Severely depressed	Effusion, RV dilation
IVC	Collapsed	Collapsed	Plethoric	Plethoric
Abdomen	Hemorrhagic free fluid	Peritoneal free fluid	—	—
Aorta	AAA, Dissection	—	—	—
Pulmonary	Normal lung sliding	Effusion, consolidation	Effusion, B-lines	Absent lung sliding

deep venous thrombosis in the lower extremity veins using bedside ultrasound adds additional evidence for the diagnosis of PE. In some cases, free-floating thrombus in the right heart may be visualized on cardiac ultrasound, and this finding is considered direct evidence of PE.[66–68]

GUIDANCE OF VOLUME MANAGEMENT

Ultrasound can help guide volume resuscitation in patients with hypotension and shock in a noninvasive manner. Traditional measures of volume status, such as CVP transduced from a central venous catheter or pulmonary capillary wedge pressure (PCWP) measured with a pulmonary artery catheter, are invasive and time consuming. CVP is known to have limited predictive value for the hemodynamic response to volume infusion,[72–74] although it is commonly used as a measure of preload in the early goal-directed therapy protocol for septic shock.[157,158] Insertion of a pulmonary artery (Swan Ganz) catheter to measure PCWP as a surrogate for left-sided filling pressures was once common in the ICU; however, studies have shown either no mortality benefit[159] or an association with increased mortality.[160] Respiratory variation in arterial pulse pressure currently has the best predictive value for hemodynamic response to volume infusion in hypotensive critically ill patients.[161,162]

Ultrasound has been proposed as a rapid, immediately available means for assessing volume status on patient presentation and to guide further fluid resuscitation during the patient's hospital course. The concept of using ultrasound to guide fluid resuscitation was introduced during the earlier discussion of IVC measurements (see **Table 1**). When seen on initial presentation of a patient in shock, a small (<1.5 cm) IVC_e that shows complete (or near complete) collapse with inspiration indicates intravascular volume depletion and aggressive fluid resuscitation should be initiated. As volume infusion proceeds, the IVC progressively increases in diameter and respiratory variation decreases. As measurements approach those seen in a plethoric IVC, a large (>2.5 cm) IVC_e that shows no (or minimal) collapse on inspiration, further volume resuscitation should be more cautious. If the patient continues to exhibit hypotension or signs of inadequate perfusion, vasopressors or ionotropes should be initiated. In such a way, serial ultrasound evaluations of the IVC, similar to trending CVP measurements, may be used to follow relative volume status and adequacy of fluid resuscitation over time.

A plethoric IVC seen on initial presentation in a patient in shock does not exclude the possibility that the patient may benefit from volume infusion.

While IVC plethora may serve as a surrogate for volume overload in cardiogenic shock, it also may be seen in obstructive etiologies of shock, when fluid resuscitation is often beneficial, as well as isolated right-sided heart failure and chronic pulmonary hypertension. Accordingly, a plethoric IVC should not be interpreted as an isolated finding, and patient care decisions should be made in light of the entire ultrasound exam as well as in the context of the patient's past medical history and current clinical presentation.

An assessment of LV function can also guide how aggressively volume should be administered in the patient in shock. Analogous to a collapsed IVC, small cardiac chamber sizes and hyperdynamic LV function suggest hypovolemic or distributive shock and safely allow for further volume expansion in most cases. On the contrary, while reduced LV function as an isolated finding does not necessarily mean that the patient's hypotension is due to cardiogenic shock or that volume infusion would be harmful, it does indicate that the patient will more quickly develop pulmonary edema if volume resuscitation is overly aggressive. If volume depletion is suspected in such patients, smaller volumes of fluid and careful reassessment after each subsequent bolus are advisable.

One proposed algorithm, the FALLS (Fluid Administration Limited by Lung Sonography) protocol, advocates continuing volume resuscitation in the hypotensive patient until early signs of pulmonary edema are recognized on pulmonary sonography.[125] It is argued that pulmonary edema and subsequent hypoxia are the major limitations to further volume resuscitation in critically ill medical patients, especially in sepsis and other distributive shock states. Since sonographic B-lines are an early sign of interstitial edema, it is proposed that their presence be used as an end point for volume resuscitation. If the critically ill patient continues to be hypotensive at this point, vasopressors or ionotropes will be necessary. The FALLS protocol may be especially useful in patients with pre-existing right-sided heart failure or pulmonary hypertension presenting with hypovolemic or distributive shock. In these patients, the IVC may appear plethoric at baseline and cannot be relied on as a reflection of effective intravascular volume status. Similarly, the FALLS protocol may also prove helpful for determining the feasibility of additional volume infusion in patients with pre-existing cardiomyopathy presenting with hypovolemic or distributive shock.

SUMMARY

An ultrasound evaluation of the critically ill patient in shock represents a new way of thinking in point-of-care ultrasound, recently acknowledged by ACEP as resuscitative ultrasound.[163] The RUSH exam serves as a standardized approach to a sonographic assessment of the unstable medical patient with undifferentiated shock. Emergency physicians and intensivists now can directly visualize a critically ill patient's underlying physiologic state of shock and rapidly exclude a number of life-threatening yet potentially reversible diagnoses, all within a matter of minutes and without ever leaving the patient's bedside. Clinicians benefit from a narrowed differential and increased confidence in the accuracy of their preliminary diagnosis. They do not have to initiate blind empiric resuscitation and instead may tailor their therapies to particular categories of shock and, in some cases, to the specific diagnosis.

While some may demand definitive studies in the literature before adopting these new technologies, many already have anecdotal experience of how bedside ultrasound can completely change a patient's course for the better.[21,23,27,164,165] Most of the individual components of the RUSH exam are familiar to clinician sonographers and have been validated for use at the patient bedside. The protocol merely serves as a structured approach incorporating multiple components into a unified whole. The intent of clinician-performed sonography is not to replace traditional methods of managing critically ill patients but to add to them. Bedside ultrasound provides an immediately available and noninvasive tool to facilitate rapid diagnosis in a multitude of life-threatening conditions. As point-of-care ultrasound continues to be embraced by clinicians in the ED and ICU, it is hoped that patients will benefit from more timely and accurate diagnoses of their underlying pathophysiology and more rapid initiation of optimal care.

REFERENCES

1. Ma OJ, Mateer JR, Ogata M, et al. Prospective analysis of a rapid trauma ultrasound examination performed by emergency physicians. J Trauma 1995;38:879–85.
2. Plummer D, Brunnette D, Asinger R, et al. Emergency department echocardiography improves outcome in penetrating cardiac injury. Ann Emerg Med 1992;21:709–12.
3. Melniker LA, Leibner E, McKenney MG, et al. Randomized controlled clinical trial of point-of-care, limited ultrasonography for trauma in the emergency department: the first sonography outcomes assessment program trial. Ann Emerg Med 2006;48:227–35.
4. Leung J, Duffy M, Finckh A. Real-time ultrasonographically-guided internal jugular vein catheterization in the emergency department increases success rates and reduces complications: a randomized, prospective study. Ann Emerg Med 2006;48:540–7.
5. Milling TJ, Rose J, Briggs WM, et al. Randomized, controlled clinical trial of point-of-care limited ultrasonography assistance of central venous cannulation: the third sonography outcomes assessment program (SOAP-3) trial. Crit Care Med 2005;33:1764–9.
6. Costantino TG, Parikh AK, Satz WA, et al. Ultrasonography-guided peripheral intravenous access versus traditional approaches in patients with difficult intravenous access. Ann Emerg Med 2005;46:456–61.
7. Nazeer SR, Dewbre H, Miller AH. Ultrasound-assisted paracentesis performed by emergency physicians vs the traditional technique: a prospective, randomized study. Am J Emerg Med 2005;23:363–7.
8. American College of Surgeons Committee on Trauma. ATLS: advance trauma life support for doctors. 8th edition. Chicago: American College of Surgeons; 2008.
9. Agency for Healthcare Research and Quality (AHRQ). Evidence Report/Technology Assessment. Number 43. Making health care safer: a critical analysis of patient safety practices. 2001. Available at: http://archive.ahrq.gov/clinic/ptsafety/pdf/front.pdf. Accessed December 27, 2010.
10. Kuhn M, Bonnin RL, Davey MJ, et al. Emergency department ultrasound scanning for abdominal aortic aneurysm: accessible, accurate, and advantageous. Ann Emerg Med 2000;36:219–23.
11. Tayal VS, Graf CD, Gibbs MA. Prospective study of accuracy and outcome of emergency ultrasound for abdominal aortic aneurysm over two years. Acad Emerg Med 2003;10:867–71.
12. Mandavia DP, Hoffner RJ, Mahaney K, et al. Bedside echocardiography by emergency physicians. Ann Emerg Med 2001;38(4):377–82.
13. Moore C, Rose GA, Tayal VS, et al. Determination of left ventricular function by emergency physician echocardiography of hypotensive patients. Acad Emerg Med 2002;9:186–93.
14. Labovitz AJ, Noble VE, Bierig M, et al. Focused cardiac ultrasound in the emergent setting: a consensus statement of the American Society of Echocardiography and American College of Emergency Physicians. J Am Soc Echocardiogr 2010;23(12):1225–30.
15. Lichtenstein D. Ultrasound in the management of thoracic disease. Crit Care Med 2007;35(Suppl 5):S250–61.
16. Volpicelli G, Silva F, Radeos M. Real-time lung ultrasound for the diagnosis of alveolar consolidation

and interstitial syndrome in the emergency department. Eur J Emerg Med 2010;17(2):63–72.

17. Moreno FL, Hagan AD, Holmen JR, et al. Evaluation of size and dynamics of the inferior vena cava as an index of right-sided cardiac function. Am J Cardiol 1984;53(4):579–85.

18. Kircher BJ, Himelman RB, Schiller NB. Noninvasive estimation of right atrial pressure from the inspiratory collapse of the inferior vena cava. Am J Cardiol 1990;66:493–6.

19. American College of Emergency Physicians Clinical Policies Committee. Clinical policy: critical issues in the evaluation and management of adult patients presenting with suspected pulmonary embolism. Ann Emerg Med 2003;41(2):257–70.

20. Lambert M, Harswick CA. Ultrasound guidance of thrombolytic therapy in pulseless electrical activity: a case report. Cal J Emerg Med 2006;7:8–11.

21. Rose JS, Bair AE, Mandavia D, et al. The UHP ultrasound protocol: a novel ultrasound approach to the empiric evaluation of the undifferentiated hypotensive patient. Am J Emerg Med 2001;19(4):299–302.

22. Jones AE, Tayal VS, Sullivan DM, et al. Randomized, controlled trial of immediate versus delayed goal-directed ultrasound to identify the cause of nontraumatic hypotension in emergency department patients. Crit Care Med 2004;32(8):1703–8.

23. Jensen MB, Sloth E, Larsen KM, et al. Transthoracic echocardiography for cardiopulmonary monitoring in intensive care. Eur J Anaesthesiol 2004;21:700–7.

24. Hernandez C, Shuler K, Hannan H, et al. C.A.U.S.E.: cardiac arrest ultra-sound exam—a better approach to managing patients in primary non-arrhythmogenic cardiac arrest. Resuscitation 2008;76(2):198–206.

25. Breitkreutz R, Price S, Steiger HV, et al. Focused echocardiographic evaluation in life support and peri-resuscitation of emergency patients: a prospective trial. Resuscitation 2010;81:1527–33.

26. Breitkreutz R, Walcher F, Seeger FH. Focused echocardiographic evaluation in resuscitation management: concept of an advanced life support-conformed algorithm. Crit Care Med 2007;35:S150–61.

27. Atkinson PRT, Mcauley DJ, Kendall RJ, et al. Abdominal and Cardiac Evaluation with Sonography in Shock (ACES): an approach by emergency physicians for the use of ultrasound in patients with undifferentiated hypotension. Emerg Med J 2009;26(2):87–91.

28. Perera P, Mailhot T, Riley D, et al. The RUSH exam: Rapid Ultrasound in SHock in the evaluation of the critically ill. Emerg Med Clin North Am 2010;28(1):29–56.

29. Weingart SD, Duque D, Nelson B. Rapid Ultrasound for Shock and Hypotension. EMedHome.com. 2010. Available at: http://www.emedhome.com/. Accessed December 7, 2010.

30. Sabia P, Abbott RD, Afrookteh A, et al. Importance of two-dimensional echocardiographic assessment of left ventricular systolic function in patients presenting to the emergency room with cardiac-related symptoms. Circulation 1991;84:1615–24.

31. Balogun MO, Omotoso AB, Bell E, et al. An audit of emergency echocardiography in a district general hospital. Int J Cardiol 1993;41:65–8.

32. Kaul S, Stratienko AA, Pollock SG, et al. Value of two-dimensional echocardiography for determining the basis of hemodynamic compromised in critically ill patients: a prospective study. J Am Soc Echocardiogr 1994;7(6):598–606.

33. Heidenreich PA, Stainback RF, Redberg RF, et al. Transesophageal echocardiography predicts mortality in critically ill patients with unexplained hypotension. J Am Coll Cardiol 1995;26(1):152–8.

34. Jones AE, Craddock PA, Tayal VS, et al. Diagnostic accuracy of left ventricular function for identifying sepsis among emergency department patients with nontraumatic symptomatic undifferentiated hypotension. Shock 2005;24(6):513–7.

35. Randazzo MR, Snoey ER, Levitt AM, et al. Accuracy of emergency physician assessment of left ventricular ejection fraction and central venous pressure using echocardiography. Acad Emerg Med 2003;10(9):973–7.

36. Gudmundsson P, Rydberg E, Winter R, et al. Visually estimated left ventricular ejection fraction by echocardiography is closely correlated with formal quantitative methods. Int J Cardiol 2005;101:209–12.

37. Mueller X, Stauffer JC, Jaussi A, et al. Subjective visual echocardiographic estimate of left ventricular ejection fraction as an alternative to conventional echocardiographic methods: comparison with contrast angiography. Clin Cardiol 1991;14:898–907.

38. Amico AF, Lichtenberg GS, Reisner SA, et al. Superiority of visual versus computerized echocardiographic estimation of radionuclide left ventricular ejection fraction. Am Heart J 1989;118:1259–65.

39. Blaivas M. Incidence of pericardial effusion in patients presenting to the emergency department with unexplained dyspnea. Acad Emerg Med 2001;8:1143–6.

40. Tayal VS, Kline JA. Emergency echocardiography to detect pericardial effusions in patients in PEA and near-PEA states. Resuscitation 2003;59:315–8.

41. Spodick DH. Acute cardiac tamponade. N Engl J Med 2003;349:684–90.

42. Larose E, Ducharne A, Mercier LA, et al. Prolonged distress and clinical deterioration before pericardial

drainage in patients with cardiac tamponade. Can J Cardiol 2000;16(3):331–6.

43. Russo AM, O'Connor WH, Waxman HL. Atypical presentations and echocardiographic findings in patients with cardiac tamponade occurring early and late after cardiac surgery. Chest 1993;104: 71–8.

44. Hauser AM. The emerging role of echocardiography in the emergency department. Ann Emerg Med 1989;18:1298–303.

45. Mayron R, Gaudio FE, Plummer D, et al. Echocardiography performed by emergency physicians: impact on diagnosis and therapy. Ann Emerg Med 1988;17:150–4.

46. Mazurek B, Jehle D, Martin M. Emergency department echocardiography in the diagnosis and therapy of cardiac tamponade. J Emerg Med 1991;9:27–31.

47. Rozycki GS, Ballard RB, Feliciano DV, et al. Surgeon-performed ultrasound for the assessment of truncal injuries: lessons learned from 1540 patients. Ann Surg 1998;39:492–8.

48. Rozycki GS, Feliciano DV, Ochsner MG, et al. The role of ultrasound in patients with possible penetrating cardiac wounds: a prospective multicenter study. J Trauma 1999;46:543–51.

49. Tsang TS, Oh JK, Seward JB, et al. Diagnostic value of echocardiography in cardiac tamponade. Herz 2000;8:734–40.

50. Armstrong WF, Schilt BF, Helper JC, et al. Diastolic collapse of the right ventricle with cardiac tamponade: an echocardiographic study. Circulation 1982;65:1491–6.

51. Gillam LD, Guyer DE, Gibson TC, et al. Hydrodynamic compression of the right atrium: a new echocardiographic sign of cardiac tamponade. Circulation 1983;68:294–301.

52. Lang RM, Bierig M, Devereux RB, et al. Recommendations for chamber quantification: a report from the American Society of Echocardiography's Guidelines and Standards Committee and the Chamber Quantification Writing Group, developed in conjunction with the European Association of Echocardiography, a branch of the European Society of Cardiology. J Am Soc Echocardiogr 2005;18(12):1440–63.

53. Rozycki GS, Feliciano FA, Schmidt JA, et al. The role of surgeon-performed ultrasound in patients with possible cardiac wounds. Ann Surg 1996; 223(6):737–46.

54. Tsang TS, Enriquez-Sarano M, Freeman WK, et al. Consecutive 1127 therapeutic echocardiographically guided pericardiocenteses: clinical profile, practice patterns, and outcomes spanning 21 years. Mayo Clin Proc 2002;77(5): 429–36.

55. Callahan JA, Seward JB, Nishimura RA, et al. Two-dimensional echocardiographically guided pericardiocentesis: experience in 117 consecutive patients. Am J Cardiol 1985;55(4):476–9.

56. Callahan JA, Seward JB. Pericardiocentesis guided by two-dimensional echocardiography. Echocardiography 1997;14(5):497–504.

57. Maggiolini S, Bozzano A, Russo P, et al. Echocardiography-guided pericardiocentesis with probe-mounted needle: report of 53 cases. J Am Soc Echocardiogr 2001;14(8):821–4.

58. Vayre F, Lardoux H, Pezzano M, et al. Subxiphoid pericardiocentesis guided by contrast two-dimensional echocardiography in cardiac tamponade: experience of 110 consecutive patients. Eur J Echocardiogr 2000;1(1):66–71.

59. Kucher N, Goldhaber SZ. Management of massive pulmonary embolism. Circulation 2005;112:e28–32.

60. Torbicki A, Perrier A, Kostantinides S, et al. Guidelines on the diagnosis and management of acute pulmonary embolism. Eur Heart J 2008;29: 2276–315.

61. Otto CM. Textbook of clinical echocardiography. 3rd edition. Philadelphia: Elsevier Saunders; 2004.

62. Nazeyrollas P, Metz D, Jolly D, et al. Use of transthoracic echocardiography combined with clinical and electrocardiographic data to predict acute pulmonary embolism. Eur Heart J 1996;17:779–86.

63. Bova C, Greco F, Misuraca G, et al. Diagnostic utility of echocardiography in patients with suspected pulmonary embolism. Am J Emerg Med 2003;21:180–3.

64. Miniati M, Monti S, Pratali L, et al. Diagnosis of pulmonary embolism: results of a prospective study in unselected patients. Am J Med 2001; 110:528–35.

65. Douglas PS, Khandheria B, Stainback RF, et al. ACCF/ASE/ACEP/ASNC/SCAI/SCCT/SCMR 2007 appropriateness criteria for transthoracic and transesophageal echocardiography. J Am Soc Echocardiogr 2007;20:787–805.

66. Konstantinides S. Acute pulmonary embolism. N Engl J Med 2008;359:2804–13.

67. Torbicki A, Galie N, Covezzoli A, et al. Right heart thrombi in pulmonary embolism. J Am Coll Cardiol 2003;42:2245–51.

68. Ferrari E, Benhamou M, Berthier F, et al. Mobile thrombi of the right heart in pulmonary embolism. Chest 2005;127:1051–3.

69. McConnell MV, Solomon SD, Rayan ME, et al. Regional right ventricular dysfunction detected by echocardiography in acute pulmonary embolism. Am J Cardiol 1996;78:469–73.

70. Lopez-Candales A, Edelman K, Candales MD. Right ventricular apical contractility in acute

pulmonary embolism: the McConnell sign revisited. Echocardiography 2010;27(6):614–20.

71. Wallace DJ, Allison M, Stone MB. Inferior vena cava percentage collapse during respiration is affected by the sampling location: an ultrasound study in healthy volunteers. Acad Emerg Med 2010;17(1):96–9.

72. Marik PE, Baram M, Vahid B. Does central venous pressure predict fluid responsiveness? A systematic review of the literature and the tale of seven mares. Chest 2008;134(1):172–8.

73. Michard F, Teboul J. Predicting fluid responsiveness in ICU patients: a critical analysis of the evidence. Chest 2002;121:2000–8.

74. Magder S, Bafaqeeh F. The clinical role of central venous pressure measurements. J Intensive Care Med 2007;22(1):44–51.

75. Ando Y, Yanagiba S, Asano Y. The inferior vena cava diameter as a marker of dry weight in chronic hemodialyzed patients. Artif Organs 1995;19: 1237–42.

76. Krause I, Birk E, Davidovits M, et al. Inferior vena cava diameter: a useful method for estimation of fluid status in children on haemodialysis. Nephrol Dial Transplant 2001;16(6):1203–6.

77. Lyon M, Blaivas M, Brannam L. Sonographic measurement of the inferior vena cava as a marker of blood loss. Am J Emerg Med 2005;23(1):45–50.

78. Yanagawa Y, Nishi K, Sakamoto T, et al. Early diagnosis of hypovolemic shock by sonographic measurement of inferior vena cava in trauma patients. J Trauma 2005;58(4):825–9.

79. Rein AJ, Lewis N, Forst L, et al. Echocardiography of the inferior vena cava in healthy subjects and in patients with cardiac disease. Isr J Med Sci 1982; 18(5):581–5.

80. Goldhammer E, Mesnick N, Abinader EG, et al. Dilated inferior vena cava: a common echocardiographic finding in highly trained elite athletes. J Am Soc Echocardiogr 1999;12:988–93.

81. Nagdev AD, Merchant RC, Tirado-Gonzalez A, et al. Emergency department bedside ultrasonographic measurement of the caval index for noninvasive determination of low central venous pressure. Ann Emerg Med 2010;55(3):290–5.

82. Ma OJ, Mateer JR, Blaivas M. Emergency ultrasound. New York: McGraw-Hill Medical; 2008.

83. Solomon SD, Bulwer BE. Essential echocardiography. Totowa (NJ): Humana Press; 2007.

84. Brennan JM, Blair JE, Goonewardena S, et al. Reappraisal of the use of inferior vena cava for estimating right atrial pressure. J Am Soc Echocardiogr 2007;20(7):857–61.

85. Blehar DJ, Dickman E, Gaspari R. Identification of congestive heart failure via respiratory variation of inferior vena cava diameter. Am J Emerg Med 2009;27(1):71–5.

86. Libby P, Braunwald E. Braunwald's heart disease: a textbook of cardiovascular medicine. 8th edition. Philadelphia: Saunders; 2008.

87. Cook DJ, Simel DL. The Rational Clinical Examination. Does this patient have abnormal central venous pressure? JAMA 1996;275(8):630–4.

88. Barbier C, Loubières Y, Schmit C, et al. Respiratory changes in inferior vena cava diameter are helpful in predicting fluid responsiveness in ventilated septic patients. Intensive Care Med 2004;30(9): 1740–6.

89. Feissel M, Michard F, Faller J-P, et al. The respiratory variation in inferior vena cava diameter as a guide to fluid therapy. Intensive Care Med 2004; 30(9):1834–7.

90. Kristensen JK, Buemann B, Kuhl E. Ultrasonic scanning in the diagnosis of splenic haematomas. Acta Chir Scand 1971;137(7):653–7.

91. Kimura A, Otsuka T. Emergency center ultrasonography in the evaluation of hemoperitoneum: a prospective study. J Trauma 1991;31(1):20–3.

92. Tso P, Rodriguez A, Cooper C, et al. Sonography in blunt abdominal trauma: a preliminary progress report. J Trauma 1992;33(1):39–43 [discussion: 43–4].

93. Jehle D, Guarino J, Karamanoukian H. Emergency department ultrasound in the evaluation of blunt abdominal trauma. Am J Emerg Med 1993;11(4): 342–6.

94. Bode PJ, Niezen RA, van Vugt AB, et al. Abdominal ultrasound as a reliable indicator for conclusive laparotomy in blunt abdominal trauma. J Trauma 1993;34(1):27–31.

95. Branney SW, Moore EE, Cantrill SV, et al. Ultrasound based key clinical pathway reduces the use of hospital resources for the evaluation of blunt abdominal trauma. J Trauma 1997;42(6): 1086–90.

96. Helling TS, Wilson J, Augustosky K. The utility of focused abdominal ultrasound in blunt abdominal trauma: a reappraisal. Am J Surg 2007;194(6): 728–32 [discussion: 732–3].

97. Hoff WS, Holevar M, Nagy KK, et al. Practice management guidelines for the evaluation of blunt abdominal trauma: the EAST practice management guidelines work group. J Trauma 2002;53(3): 602–15.

98. American College of Radiology. ACR-AIUM Practice Guideline for the Performance of an Ultrasound Examination of the Abdomen and/or Retroperitoneum. 2007. Revised. Available at: http://www.acr.org/SecondaryMainMenuCategories/quality_safety/guidelines/us/us_abdomen_retro.aspx. Accessed December 20, 2010.

99. Atri M, Valenti DA, Bret PM, et al. Effect of transvaginal sonography on the use of invasive procedures for evaluating patients with a clinical

diagnosis of ectopic pregnancy. J Clin Ultrasound 2003;22(4):409–10.

100. Von Kuenssberg Jehle D, Stiller G, Wagner D. Sensitivity in detecting free intraperitoneal fluid with the pelvic views of the FAST exam. Am J Emerg Med 2003;21:476–8.

101. Noble VE, Nelson B, Sutingco AN. Manual of emergency and critical care ultrasound. New York: Cambridge University Press; 2007.

102. Tiling T, Bouillon B, Schmid A, et al. Ultrasound in blunt abdomino-thoracic trauma. In: Border JR, Allgoewer M, Hansen ST, et al, editors. Blunt multiple trauma: comprehensive pathophysiology and care. New York: Marcel Dekker; 1990. p. 415–33.

103. Branney SW, Wolfe RE, Moore EE, et al. Quantitative sensitivity of ultrasound in detecting free intraperitoneal fluid. J Trauma 1995;39(2):375–80.

104. Sisley AC, Rozycki GS, Ballard RB, et al. Rapid detection of traumatic effusions using surgeon-performed ultrasonography. J Trauma 1998;44(2):291–6.

105. Ma OJ, Mateer JR. Trauma ultrasound vs chest radiography in the detection of hemothorax. Ann Emerg Med 1997;29(3):312–5.

106. Rowan KR, Kirkpatrick AW, Liu D, et al. Traumatic pneumothorax detection with US: correlation with chest radiography and CT–initial experience. Radiology 2002;225(1):210–4.

107. Lederle FA, Simel DL. Does this patient have abdominal aortic aneurysm? JAMA 1999;281: 77–82.

108. Fink HA, Lederle FA, Roth CS, et al. The accuracy of physical examination to detect abdominal aortic aneurysm. Arch Intern Med 2000;160(6):833–6.

109. Plummer D, Clinton J, Matthew B. Emergency department ultrasound improves time to diagnosis and survival of abdominal aortic aneurysm. Acad Emerg Med 1998;5:417.

110. Ernst CB. Abdominal aortic aneurysm. N Engl J Med 1993;328(16):1167–72.

111. Dent B, Kendall RJ, Boyle AA, et al. Emergency ultrasound of the abdominal aorta by UK emergency physicians: a prospective cohort study. Emerg Med J 2007;24:547–9.

112. Costantino TG, Bruno EC, Handly N, et al. Accuracy of emergency medicine ultrasound in the evaluation of abdominal aortic aneurysm. J Emerg Med 2005;29:455–60.

113. Knaut AL, Kendall JL, Patten R, et al. Ultrasonographic measurement of aortic diameter by emergency physicians approximates results obtained by computed tomography. J Emerg Med 2005;28: 119–26.

114. Fleming C, Whitlock EP, Beil TL, et al. Screening for abdominal aortic aneurysm: a best-evidence systematic review for the U.S. Preventive Services Task Force. Ann Intern Med 2005;142:203–11.

115. Han SS, Huang RR. Results of 101 ruptured abdominal aortic aneurysm repairs from a single surgical practice. Arch Surg 2003;138:898–901.

116. Harris LM, Faggioli GL, Fiedler R, et al. Ruptured abdominal aortic aneurysms: factors affecting mortality rates. J Vasc Surg 1991;14:812–8.

117. Daily P, Trueblood H, Stinson, et al. Management of acute aortic dissections. Ann Thorac Surg 1970;10: 237–47.

118. Miller D. Surgical management of aortic dissections: indications, peri-operative management and long term results. In: Doroghazi RM, Slater EE, editors. Aortic dissection. New York: McGraw-Hill; 1983. p. 193–243.

119. Appelbaum A, Karp R, Kirklin J. Ascending vs descending aortic dissections. Ann Surg 1976;183: 296–300.

120. Meredith EL, Masani ND. Echocardiography in the emergency assessment of acute aortic syndromes. Eur J Echocardiogr 2009;10:i31–9.

121. Blaivas M, Theodoro D. Frequency of incomplete abdominal aorta visualization by emergency department bedside ultrasound. Acad Emerg Med 2004;11(1):103–5.

122. Moore CL, Holliday RS, Hwang JQ, et al. Screening for abdominal aortic aneurysm in asymptomatic at-risk patients using emergency ultrasound. Am J Emerg Med 2008;26:883–7.

123. Braunwald E. Harrison's principles of internal medicine. 15th edition. New York: McGraw-Hill; 2001.

124. Middleton WD, Kurtz AB, Hertzberg BS. Ultrasound: the requisites. 2nd edition. St Louis (MO): Mosby; 2004.

125. Lichtenstein DA. Whole body ultrasonography in the critically ill. New York: Springer; 2010.

126. Blaivas M, Lyon M, Duggal S. A prospective comparison of supine chest radiography and bedside ultrasound for the diagnosis of traumatic pneumothorax. Acad Emerg Med 2005;12(9):844–9.

127. Lichtenstein DA, Mezière G, Lascols N, et al. Ultrasound diagnosis of occult pneumothorax. Crit Care Med 2005;33(6):1231–8.

128. Wilkerson RG, Stone MB. Sensitivity of bedside ultrasound and supine anteroposterior chest radiographs for the identification of pneumothorax after blunt trauma. Acad Emerg Med 2010;17(1):11–7.

129. Soldati G, Testa A, Sher S, et al. Occult traumatic pneumothorax: diagnostic accuracy of lung ultrasonography in the emergency department. Chest 2008;133:204–11.

130. Lichtenstein D, Mezière G, Biderman P, et al. The "lung point": an ultrasound sign specific to pneumothorax. Intensive Care Med 2000;26(10): 1434–40.

131. Slater A, Goodwin M, Anderson K, et al. COPD can mimic the appearance of pneumothorax on thoracic ultrasound. Chest 2006;129(3):545.

132. Blaivas M, Tsung JW. Point-of-care sonographic detection of left endobronchial main stem intubation and obstruction versus endotracheal intubation. J Ultrasound Med 2008;27(5):785–9.

133. Chun R, Kirkpatrick A, Sirois M, et al. Where's the tube? Evaluation of hand-held ultrasound in confirming endotracheal tube placement. Prehospital Disaster Med 2004;19(4):366–9.

134. Lichtenstein D, Mézière G, Biderman P, et al. The comet-tail artifact. An ultrasound sign of alveolar-interstitial syndrome. Am J Respir Crit Care Med 1997;156(5):1640–6.

135. Lichtenstein D, Mezière G, Biderman P, et al. The comet-tail artifact: an ultrasound sign ruling out pneumothorax. Intensive Care Med 1999;25(4):383–8.

136. Agricola E, Bove T, Oppizzi M, et al. "Ultrasound comet-tail images": a marker of pulmonary edema: a comparative study with wedge pressure and extravascular lung water. Chest 2005;127(5):1690–5.

137. Soldati G, Copetti R, Sher S. Sonographic interstitial syndrome: the sound of lung water. J Ultrasound Med 2009;28(2):163–74.

138. Volpicelli G, Cardinale L, Garofalo G, et al. Usefulness of lung ultrasound in the bedside distinction between pulmonary edema and exacerbation of COPD. Emerg Radiol 2008;15:145–51.

139. Soldati G, Sher S. Bedside lung ultrasound in critical care practice. Minerva Anestesiol 2009;75:509–17.

140. Volpicelli G, Caramello V, Cardinale L, et al. Bedside ultrasound of the lung for the monitoring of acute decompensated heart failure. Am J Emerg Med 2008;26:585–91.

141. Copetti R, Soldati G, Copetti P. Chest sonography: a useful tool to differentiate acute cardiogenic pulmonary edema from acute respiratory distress syndrome. Cardiovasc Ultrasound 2008;6:16.

142. Noble VE, Murray AF, Capp R, et al. Ultrasound assessment for extravascular lung water in patients undergoing hemodialysis: time course for resolution. Chest 2009;135:1433–9.

143. Liteplo AS, Marill KA, Villen T, et al. Emergency thoracic ultrasound in the differentiation of the etiology of shortness of breath (ETUDES): sonographic B-lines and N-terminal pro-brain-type natriuretic peptide in diagnosing congestive heart failure. Acad Emerg Med 2009;16(3):201–10.

144. Volpicelli G, Noble V, Liteplo A, et al. Decreased sensitivity of lung ultrasound limited to the anterior chest in emergency department diagnosis of cardiogenic pulmonary edema: a retrospective analysis. Crit Ultrasound J 2010;2(2):47–52.

145. Cardinale L, Volpicelli G, Binello F, et al. Clinical application of lung ultrasound in patients with acute dyspnea: differential diagnosis between cardiogenic and pulmonary causes. Radiol Med 2009;114:1053–64.

146. Volpicelli G, Cardinale L, Mussa A, et al. Diagnosis of cardiogenic pulmonary edema limited to the anterior lung. Chest 2009;135:883.

147. Volpicelli G, Caramello V, Cardinale L, et al. Detection of sonographic B-lines in patients with normal lung or radiographic alveolar consolidation. Med Sci Monit 2008;14(3):CR122–8.

148. Reissig A, Kroegel C. Transthoracic sonography of diffuse parenchymal lung disease: the role of comet tail artifacts. J Ultrasound Med 2003;22:173–80.

149. Volpicelli G, Mussa A, Garofalo G, et al. Bedside lung ultrasound in the assessment of alveolar-interstitial syndrome. Am J Emerg Med 2006;24(6):689–96.

150. Volpicelli G, Frascisco M. Sonographic detection of radio-occult interstitial lung involvement in measles pneumonitis. Am J Emerg Med 2009;27(1):128.

151. Peris A, Zagli G, Barbani F, et al. The value of lung ultrasound monitoring in H1N1 acute respiratory distress syndrome. Anaesthesia 2010;65:294–7.

152. Via G, Lichtenstein D, Mojoli F, et al. Whole lung lavage: a unique model for ultrasound assessment of lung aeration changes. Intensive Care Med 2010;36(6):999–1007.

153. Lichtenstein DA, Lascols N, Meziere G, et al. Ultrasound diagnosis of alveolar consolidation in the critically ill. Intensive Care Med 2004;30:276–81.

154. Yu C-J, Yang P-C, Chang D-B, et al. Diagnostic and therapeutic use of chest sonography: value in critically ill patients. Am J Roentgenol 1992;159(4):695–701.

155. Lichtenstein D, Goldstein I, Mourgeon E, et al. Comparative diagnostic performance of auscultation, chest radiography, and lung ultrasonography in acute respiratory distress syndrome. Anesthesiology 2004;100:9–15.

156. Grimberg A, Shigueoka DC, Atallah AN, et al. Diagnostic accuracy of sonography for pleural effusion: systematic review. Sao Paulo Med J 2010;128(2):90–5.

157. Rivers E, Hguyen B, Havstad S, et al. Early goal-directed therapy in the treatment of severe sepsis and septic shock. N Engl J Med 2001;345(19):1368–77.

158. Dellinger R, Levy M, Carlet J, et al. Surviving Sepsis Campaign: international guidelines for management of severe sepsis and septic shock. Crit Care Med 2008;2008:296–327.

159. Yu DT, Platt R, Lanken PN, et al. Relationship of pulmonary artery catheter use to mortality and resource utilization in patients with severe sepsis. Crit Care Med 2003;31:2734–41.

160. Connors AF, Speroff T, Dawson NV, et al. The effectiveness of right heart catheterization in the initial care of critically ill patients. JAMA 1996;276(11):889–97.

161. Michard F, Boussat S, Chelma D, et al. Relation between respiratory changes in arterial pulse

pressure and fluid responsiveness in septic patients with acute circulatory failure. Am J Respir Crit Care Med 2000;162:134–8.

162. Tavernier B, Makhotine O, Lebuffe G, et al. Systolic pressure variation as a guide to fluid therapy in patients with sepsis-induced hypotension. Anesthesiology 1998;89:1309–10.

163. American College of Emergency Physicians. Policy statement: emergency ultrasound guidelines. Ann Emerg Med 2009;53:550–70.

164. Dean AJ. Bedside ultrasound as an adjunct in the evaluation of critically ill patients. In: Brooks A, Connolly J, Chan O, editors. Ultrasound in emergency care. Malden (MA): Blackwell Publishing; 2004. p. 59–75.

165. Hendrickson RG, Dean AJ, Costantino TG. A novel use of ultrasound in pulseless electrical activity: the diagnosis of an acute abdominal aortic aneurysm rupture. J Emerg Med 2001; 21(2):141–4.

The Rapid Assessment of Dyspnea with Ultrasound: RADiUS

William Manson, MD*, Nadim Mike Hafez, MD

KEYWORDS

- Emergency • Ultrasound • Dyspnea • Critical care

This article reviews the focused bedside ultrasonography examination performed to evaluate the patient who presents with undifferentiated dyspnea. This 4-step ultrasonographic protocol combines cardiac and thoracic ultrasonography applications into 1 focused examination. The authors refer to this new ultrasonographic protocol as the rapid assessment of dyspnea with ultrasonography (RADiUS). This protocol involves multiple limited examinations, including echocardiography and evaluation of the thoracic cavity.

Many emergency and critical care physicians are already performing the components of this examination as a part of their daily practice through the use of both the FAST (focused assessment with sonography in trauma) examination[1] and RUSH (rapid ultrasonography in shock) protocol.[2,3] In the mid-90s, the FAST examination became an important tool in the rapid evaluation of the patient with trauma. This examination combined a limited evaluation for free intra-abdominal fluid with the assessment of pericardial effusion. Although it involved only 4 limited views, this clinician-performed ultrasonographic evaluation at the point of care revolutionized the care of the acutely injured patient, by identifying critical patients needing emergent laparotomy. The FAST examination has recently been expanded to the Extended FAST (E-FAST)[4] examination through the addition of pneumothorax evaluation. More recently, the RUSH protocol developed the concept of resuscitation ultrasonography with its 3-step protocol. This examination intends to provide the clinician with a more accurate initial diagnosis in patients presenting with undifferentiated hypotension. The RUSH protocol combines limited echocardiography, the EFAST, limited aorta, and focused inferior vena cava (IVC) evaluation.

The RADiUS examination involves 4 different components. These include (1) a focused cardiac examination, (2) a focused IVC evaluation, (3) evaluation of the thoracic cavity for pleural effusions, and (4) assessment of the pleural line. The physician may also choose to include a focused assessment of the lower extremities for deep venous thrombosis (DVT). However, this examination is time consuming and may not be required for all patients.

The cardiac portion of the examination is considered the most technically challenging because the examiner needs to image the cardiac structures from multiple different scan planes. The cardiac portion of the examination evaluates for presence of pericardial effusion, and it also assesses left ventricular function and right ventricular dilation indicating right ventricular strain. This portion also allows the sonologist to evaluate the patient's intravascular volume and response to fluid resuscitation. The sonographic evaluation for the presence of pleural effusions is easily performed and typically is straightforward. This assessment can be performed in a supine patient in a similar fashion to the hepatorenal and splenorenal views of the FAST examination. The pleural evaluation can assess for pneumothorax and presence of interstitial fluid.

The authors have nothing to disclose.
There was no funding for this project.
Department of Emergency Medicine, Emory University School of Medicine, 49 Jesse Hill Jr Drive, Atlanta, GA 30303, USA
* Corresponding author.
E-mail address: wmanson@emory.edu

Ultrasound Clin 6 (2011) 261–276
doi:10.1016/j.cult.2011.03.010

Similar to the timing of the FAST examination, which may occur at the end of the primary survey or during the secondary survey, there are no hard rules for when the physician should perform the RADiUS examination. The examination should complement, not replace, a focused history and physical examination. The RADiUS examination should never delay treatment of an emergent airway, but aids the physician in the subsequent management of the critically ill patient (**Fig. 1**).

CARDIAC ULTRASONOGRAPHIC EXAMINATION

The evaluation of the patient's heart can provide more information than any other aspect of the

RADiUS examination, but is also the most challenging component of the evaluation. Comprehensive echocardiography, typically performed by sonographers and interpreted by dedicated cardiologists, is not routinely available in most emergency departments. A study by Moore and colleagues[5] in 2006 noted that 26% of emergency departments had no accesses to formal echocardiography and only 29% had 24-hour availability of echocardiography within their institution. Given this lack of immediate availability of echocardiology, it is not surprising that focused cardiac ultrasonography has now become a standard component of the emergent evaluation of patients with acute cardiopulmonary disease and of emergency medicine training.[6,7]

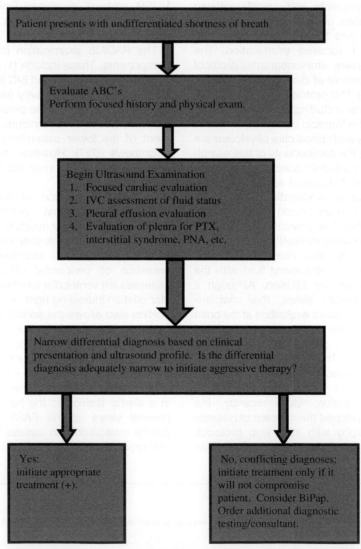

Fig. 1. Ultrasound evaluation of patient presenting with undifferentiated dyspnea. This flow diagram proposes an integration of the RADiUS examination into the clinical evaluation of a patient. ABCs, airway, breathing, and circulation; BiPAP, bilevel positive airway pressure; PNA, pneumonia; PTX, pneumothorax.

Box 1
High-risk populations for pericardial effusion

1. Unexplained dyspnea or hypotension
2. Cancer with chest pain or dyspnea
3. Congestive heart failure (CHF)/enlarged cardiac silhouette
4. Blunt chest injury
5. Penetrating chest injury
6. Uremia with chest pain or dyspnea
7. Pericarditis
8. Systemic lupus erythematosis with chest pain or dyspnea

Data from Mandavia D, Hoffner R, Mahaney K, et al. Bedside echocardiography by emergency physicians. Ann Emerg Med 2001;38(4):377–82.

The benefit of brief cardiac ultrasonography by the treating physician has been noted by several investigators. A study in 1989 by Hauser[8] noted the list of potential diseases that an emergency physician could diagnose with a brief ultrasonography of the heart, including cardiogenic shock, cardiac tamponade, pulmonary embolism (PE), and ischemia. Another study by Kimura and colleagues[9] in 2001 noted the potential benefit of performing a brief screening cardiac ultrasonography on patients in a chest pain center. This study compared brief cardiac ultrasonography of the parasternal long-axis view with a comprehensive formal echocardiographic examination. The examinations were performed by a cardiologist or an experienced cardiac sonographer, and later formally interpreted by a cardiologist. In a small subset of patients, nonphysician personnel from the emergency department also performed screening ultrasonography. The study noted a clear benefit to identifying significant cardiac

disease, even if the sensitivity of the screening examination did not match that of the comprehensive echocardiogram. More recently, the American College of Emergency Physicians and the American Society of Echocardiography have written a joint paper highlighting the benefits of focused bedside echocardiography.[10]

Pericardial Effusion

Several studies have shown that noncardiologist physicians are capable of accurately identifying pericardial effusions with focused cardiac sonography. In 2001, Mandavia and colleagues[11] published one of the first studies assessing the accuracy of trained emergency physicians in correctly diagnosing pericardial effusions. Trained emergency physicians performed a focused cardiac ultrasonographic examination on 515 patients deemed at high risk for pericardial effusion based on their medical history and presenting symptoms (**Box 1**). Review of the scans by a cardiologist with expertise in echocardiography noted sensitivity of 96% and a specificity of 98% for the diagnosis of a pericardial effusion, with 93% of the 515 patients examined having technically adequate scans. The positive predictive value (PPV) was 92.5% and the negative predictive value (NPV) was 98.8%. In addition, Tayal and Kline[12] published a small study in 2003 reporting that goal-directed emergency physician echocardiography performed on patients with pulseless electrical activity allowed for the identification of underlying life-threatening pathologies as well as the rapid initiation of correcting treatments.

When identifying pericardial effusion, emergency physicians and surgeons are typically comfortable with the subcostal view (**Fig. 2**), which is a routine part of the FAST examination.[1]

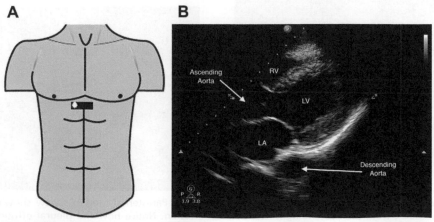

Fig. 2. (*A*) Subxiphoid view probe position. (*B*) Normal subxiphoid view. LA, left atrium; LV, left ventricle; RA, right atrium; RV, right ventricle.

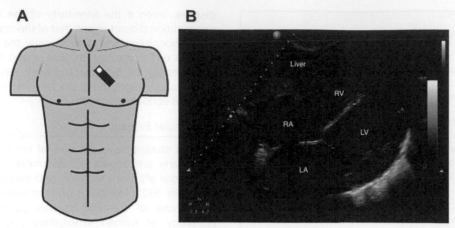

Fig. 3. (*A*) Parasternal long view probe position. (*B*) Normal parasternal long axis. LA, left atrium; LV, left ventricle; RV, right ventricle.

However, almost any cardiac view is capable of identifying large pericardial effusions. The parasternal long-axis view (see **Fig. 3**) is particularly helpful in differentiating pericardial effusion from pleural effusion. In this view, a pericardial effusion appears as an anechoic space in the far field of the image. It is located posterior to the left ventricle/left atrium, but anterior to the descending aorta (**Fig. 4**).[13] In contrast, a pleural effusion is seen as an anechoic area tracking posterior to the aorta (**Fig. 5**).

Quantifying pericardial effusion can also be performed at the bedside. Small effusions exist when separation between the heart and parietal pericardium is less than 0.5 cm. Moderate effusions are 0.5 cm to 2 cm, and large effusion are greater than 2 cm.[13] However, other studies have reported different values. A 2001 study by Blaivas[14] using

subcostal and parasternal views defined large effusions as greater than 15 mm and small effusions as less than 10 mm.

Cardiac Tamponade

Although the size of pericardial effusion does not predict tamponade physiology, the rate of accumulation of the effusion often determines whether a patient develops tamponade. Some patients with tamponade physiology can be identified by Beck's triad of hypotension, jugular venous distension, and distant, muffled heart sounds on physical examination. However, these signs are frequently absent in all patients with significant pericardial effusions and tamponade.[15] As pericardial pressure rises in tamponade, the right ventricle may begin to collapse during diastole, suggesting

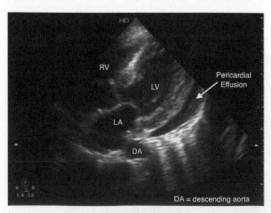

Fig. 4. Parasternal long-axis view showing a pericardial effusion. Notice how the pericardial effusion separates the heart from the descending aorta. DA, descending aorta; LA, left atrium; LV, left ventricle; RV, right ventricle.

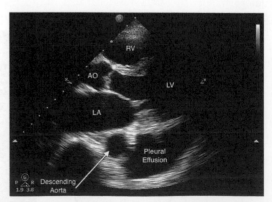

Fig. 5. Parasternal long-axis view showing a pleural effusion. Notice how the pleural effusion is located distal to the descending aorta. AO, ascending aorta; LA, left atrium; LV, left ventricle; RV, right ventricle.

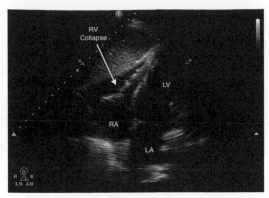

Fig. 6. Subxiphoid view showing a pericardial effusion between the liver and right ventricle (RV). The collapse of the RV during diastole indicates tamponade physiology. LA, left atrium; LV, left ventricle; RA, right atrium.

pericardial tamponade (**Box 9, Fig. 6**). In addition, the thin-walled right atrium may begin to collapse during systole (**Fig. 7**).[13]

Left Ventricular Function

Although precise quantification of left ventricular dysfunction is clearly better suited to cardiologists, assessment of the quality of left ventricular function can often be assessed on focused cardiac sonography. In 2002, Moore and colleagues[16] noted that appropriately trained emergency physicians using only visual qualitative estimation of left ventricular function could accurately assess the degree of left ventricular dysfunction when compared with formal echocardiographic calculations. The interobserver variability between the primary cardiologist and the emergency physicians (Pearson correlation coefficient $R = 0.86$) determination of left ventricular function compared favorably with the interobserver variability between cardiologists ($R = 0.84$). Previous studies

evaluating cardiologists' visual estimation of ejection fraction have shown similar levels of correlation ($R = 0.77$–0.90).[17,18]

Other studies have shown similar results. Randazzo and colleagues[19] in 2003 also reported that emergency physicians and cardiologists agree with regards to qualitative assessment of left ventricular function. Their study, which enrolled more than 100 patients, noted excellent agreement (86%) between cardiologists and emergency physicians. In 2009, Melamed and colleagues[20] reported that intensivists with minimal goal-directed training had similar success.

PE

Although the sensitivity of echocardiography to detect patients with acute PE ranges from 40% to 70%,[13] the examination has been shown to have a high specificity for PE when right ventricular hypokinesis with apical sparing is noted.[21] On sonographic examination the right ventricle shows significantly decreased function, but the apex of the right ventricle shows motion similar to a normal heart (**Box 2, Fig. 8**). This sign, first described by McConnell in 1996 and now know as the McConnell sign, has 94% specificity and an NPV of 96%. A recent case study by Bomann and Moore[22] showed the value of this finding when it led emergency physicians to diagnose and save an unstable patient through thrombolytic therapy.

Some investigators have attempted to combine clinical findings with echocardiographic data to diagnose PE. A European study in 1996 attempted to combine clinical findings (hepatojugular reflux, signs of DVT, and S1-Q3 on EKG) and echocardiographic parameters from patients with a suspected PE.[23] This combination resulted in a sensitivity of 96% and specificity of 83% for the presence of a PE. However, this study was limited by broad exclusion criteria, incomplete patient data, and a small sample size. Grifoni and colleagues[24] in

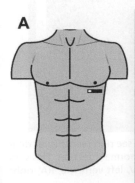

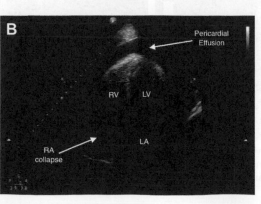

Fig. 7. (A) Apical 4-chamber view probe position. (B) Apical 4-chamber view showing a large pericardial effusion and collapse of the right atrium (RA) during systole, indicating tamponade physiology. The right atrium is scalloped inward in a concave arc, opposed to the normal convex shape of the right atrium. LA, left atrium; LV, left ventricle; RV, right ventricle.

Mansencal and colleagues[25] in 2008 combined echocardiography and DVT evaluation in patients with a positive D-dimer screening test. In their high-risk population, they generated only 87% combined sensitivity and 69% specificity. However, this concept may prove valuable in the future, because no one has studied the effect of using the Well's criteria **Box 3** or the PE rule-out criteria **Box 4** in combination with bedside echocardiography to exclude PE.[26,27]

ULTRASOUND EXAMINATION OF THE IVC

Evaluation of intravascular fluid status is a necessary but challenging component of treating patients with dyspnea or hypotension. Vital signs and physical examination findings too often fail to reliably assess the patient's volume status. More invasive means of obtaining these data are available but require extensive procedures and specialized equipment not readily available to all physicians. Ultrasound examination of the IVC is a noninvasive, reliable, and repeatable alternative that can be used to differentiate between a physiologic state of fluid overload or

1998 combined echocardiography, clinical features, and a lower extremity duplex ultrasonography to identify patients with PE. These investigators reported a sensitivity of only 89% and specificity of 74%. A more recent study by

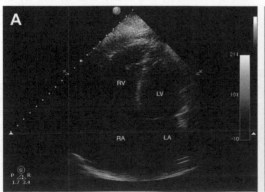 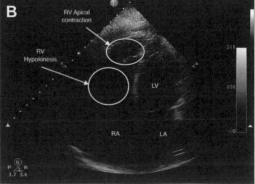

Fig. 8. (A, B) Apical 4-chamber view showing a positive McConnell sign. In this view we see right ventricular dilation (RV/LV ratio >1:1) and hypokinesis. However, the apex of the right ventricle shows normal function. This sign has a 94% specificity for pulmonary embolus and an NPV of 96%.[20] LA, left atrium; LV, left ventricle; RA, right atrium.

Box 4
PE rule-out criteria

- Age less than 50 years
- Heart rate less than 100 bpm
- Oxygen saturation on room air greater than 94%
- No previous DVT/PE
- No recent trauma or surgery
- No hemoptysis
- No exogenous estrogen
- No clinical signs suggesting DVT

Table 1
Estimation of right atrial pressure (RAP)

IVC Diameter (cm)	% Change with Respiration	Estimated RAP
<1.2	Spontaneous collapse	Volume depletion
<1.7	>50%	0–5 mm Hg
>1.7	>50%	5–10 mm Hg
>1.7	<50%	10–15 mm Hg
>1.7	No change	15–20 mm Hg
Dilated with dilated hepatic veins	No change	>20 mm Hg

one of intravascular fluid depletion. Earlier work by cardiologists has focused on an assessment of the diameter of the IVC in conjunction with its variation throughout spontaneous respiration to estimate right atrial pressure.[28,29] **Table 1** summarizes these findings from the American Society of Echocardiography. A study by Randazzo and colleagues[15] showed that assessment of the central venous pressure by point-of-care physicians correlated 83.3% of the time with the formal assessment of the same ultrasonographic images by a staff cardiologist.

Collapsibility of the IVC is an excellent predictor of a patient's volume status. Greater than 50% collapse of the IVC with spontaneous respiration **Fig. 18** correlates best with intravascular volume depletion.[29,30] Some investigators advocate the use of M-mode to help determine the size variations of the vessels with respiration, but this may result in inaccurate measurements secondary to caudal displacement of the IVC during spontaneous respirations.[31] Many attempts have been made to identify alternative ultrasonographic markers of intravascular volume status. Dilation of the IVC diameter in short axis greater than 10 mm has been proposed as the cutoff for identifying fluid overload.[32] Given the variation in estimations of measurements/volumes among the various studies, Wallace and colleagues[31] attempted to standardize the location to measure the IVC to

ensure reproducibility between patients and physicians. These investigators concluded that the most consistent locations for measuring IVC collapse are (1) the IVC in transverse view at the level of the left renal vein and (2) the longitudinal view of the IVC through the liver, 2 cm caudal to the hepatic vein inlet. In addition, some researchers have gone beyond traditional methods and have used peripheral venous-compression ultrasonography as well as an ultrasonographic evaluation of the internal jugular vein to evaluate the intravascular volume status. However, these techniques require additional research before they are validated.[33,34]

Although only a binary examination, the evaluation of IVC collapsibility can rapidly narrow the differential diagnosis. Right ventricular dilation in the presence of a plethoric IVC **(Fig. 9)** may indicate right heart failure, PE, or pulmonary hypertension. A dilated IVC may also be present in cardiac tamponade or long-standing left ventricular dysfunction. Patients in sepsis may present with intravascular volume depletion and hyperdynamic cardiac activity. For patients with presumed COPD

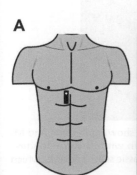 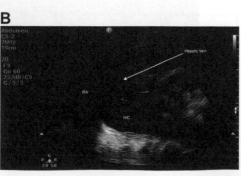

Fig. 9. (*A*) IVC view probe position. (*B*) IVC as it enters the right atrium (RA). The hepatic vein is also visible and can be seen communicating with the IVC. Both the IVC as well as the hepatic vein are fully dilated. A plethoric IVC may be consistent with increases in intravascular volume or increased right heart pressures.

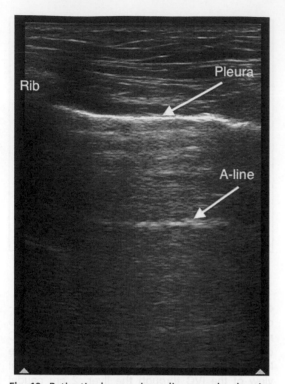

Fig. 10. Patient's pleura using a linear probe showing an A-line artifact. A-lines are a type of reverberation artifact that is the result of ultrasound beams reflecting off the pleura. These lines appear at equal distances, distal from the original signal of the pleura. When A-lines are present in the absence of B-lines they suggest that interstitial edema is not present.

exacerbation, IVC volume status may vary, and its effects on the patients' symptoms have to be interpreted in light of the presence or absence of various comorbidities.

ULTRASOUND EXAMINATION OF THE LUNGS AND PLEURA

The ultrasonographic assessment of the lungs in a patient with undifferentiated shortness of breath can yield a significant amount of information regarding a wide variety of clinical conditions. These results should be interpreted in context of the previous examinations of both the heart and the IVC when making clinical decisions. Ultrasound of the pleura is capable of identifying a pneumothorax, interstitial edema, acute respiratory distress syndrome (ARDS), noncardiogenic pulmonary edema, and consolidation. Imaging the thoracic cavity above the diaphragm allows for the identification of a pleural effusion or hemothorax that is not visible on chest radiograph.

Ultrasound is more sensitive and specific than chest radiography for detection of pneumothorax in all patients.[35] Normal lung tissue on ultrasonography is characterized by the presence of a hyperechoic pleural line with pleural movement (lung sliding) and multiple reverberation artifacts know as A-lines. These artifacts are hyperechoic lines that are present distal to the pleural line, arising at equal distances. The reverberation artifact is created by high difference in tissue density around the pleural line caused by subpleural air (**Fig. 10**). A pneumothorax can be diagnosed on sonography by showing the absence of lung sliding, the absence of the comet-tail artifact, and/or the presence of a lung point.[36–38] Traditional examination of the lung to detect pneumothorax is performed in B-mode or M-mode (**Fig. 11**) but some investigators have advocated the use of power Doppler.[4] This technology detects movements at low velocities and can highlight the subtle

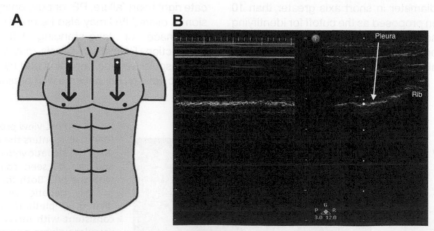

Fig. 11. (*A*) Probe position for pleural evaluation. (*B*) Split-screen image of the pleura, showing B-mode and M-mode simultaneously. The right side shows the hyperechoic pleura and the adjacent rib with its corresponding shadow in B mode. The left side shows the corresponding M-mode image with the classic seashore sign, which indicates normal lung motion and hence the absence of a pneumothorax.

movements of the pleura. In the setting of a pneumothorax the power Doppler signal highlighting the pleural movement is absent. Other investigators have cautioned about sole reliance on the absence of lung sliding, as the sole objective for diagnosing lung collapse, because this finding can be common in right main stem intubations, lung consolidations, and any other process that separates the visceral and parietal pleura.[39] The specificity of lung sliding ranges from 91% to 100%. The sensitivity of lung sliding to detect pneumothorax ranges from 95% to 100%.[35,40–42] These numbers vary largely depending on the number of lung fields examined. The sensitivity of finding a small pneumothorax increases with the number of lung fields examined.

Several other sonographic findings other than lung sliding may aid in the diagnosis of pneumothorax (**Box 5**; **Fig. 12**). Comet-tail artifacts, another type of reverberation artifact, originating at the pleural line, are usually present in normal lung tissue. Comet-tail artifacts differ from A-lines in that they arise from the pleural line as a hyperechoic tail, directed perpendicularly away from the pleural line (**Fig. 13**). Although comet-tail

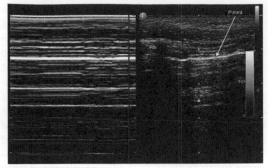

Fig. 12. Split-screen image of B-mode on the right and M-mode on the left. This image shows the pleural line in the B-mode image, with a rib and its shadow at the edge of the image. The M-mode tracing lacks the sandy appearance distal to the pleural line. Instead, horizontal hyperechoic lines extend beyond the pleural line. This image shows the stratosphere sign, indicating a pneumothorax. Contrast this image with **Fig. 11** (seashore sign).

artifacts are absent in almost all cases of pneumothorax, they are only 60% specific for the diagnosis of pneumothorax. A combination of absent lung sliding and absent comet-tail artifacts

---

Box 5
Case 3

- Clinical History
  - An 18-year-old female patient presented with pleuritic right chest, shoulder pain, and shortness of breath for 12 hours. She denied any family history of PE, coronary artery disease (CAD), or coagulopathy. She denied taking any medications including oral contraceptive pills. She was currently on her menstrual period. She was tachypneic, tachycardic, and her pulse oximetry was 94% on room air, but had an otherwise unremarkable clinical examination.

- Findings
  - The RADiUS examination revealed the following information: parasternal long and apical 4-chamber views show no normal left ventricular function; the IVC was normal in size and varied less than 50% with spontaneous respiration; examination of the right pleura showed stratosphere sign on M-mode (see **Fig. 12**); examination for effusion on the right side showed loss of mirror-image artifact.

- Diagnosis
  - The RADiUS examination confirmed the diagnosis of catamenial pneumothorax.

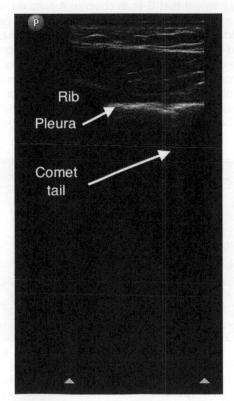

Fig. 13. Patient's pleura showing the comet-tail artifact arising from the pleural line. Comet-tails are a type of reverberation artifact that are seen coming from the pleura line in normal individuals.

improves diagnostic accuracy and has been shown to have 100% sensitivity and 96.5% specificity.[37] Lichtenstein and colleagues[38] introduced the concept of a lung point to describe the transition point in the thorax between the normal pleura and pneumothorax. These investigators identified the point where the visceral and parietal pleura separated, indicating the beginning of the pneumothorax. The presence of a lung point was found to be 66% sensitive and 100% specific. Lichtenstein and Meziere[43] combined these findings to yield a sensitivity of 88% and a specificity of 100% with a PPV of 100% and an NPV of 99%.

Evaluation of the pleural line artifacts can differentiate between some of the most common conditions encountered in critical patients.[43,44] A-lines are a reverberation artifact of the pleural line; they are present in normal lungs and are often more prominent in patients with COPD and asthma (see Fig. 10). B-lines are a type of comet-tail artifact arising from the pleural line; they are hyperechoic reverberations that move with lung sliding and extend the length of the viewing screen (Fig. 14). More specific definitions have been proposed by various investigators, including the requirement that B-lines obscure A-lines on real-time imaging, but these findings have not been validated.[43] B-lines represent extravascular lung fluid or any process that increases the normal size of the interlobular pulmonary septae, including fibrosis or infection.[45,46] Both the distribution and number of B-lines help to differentiate various disease processes. Unilateral B-lines are believed to be consistent with an inflammatory process

such as pneumonia. B-lines associated with a pulmonary contusion carry a sensitivity of 94.6% and specificity of 96.1%.[47] When assessing patients with dyspnea in the intensive care unit (ICU), the predominance of B-lines on one side of the chest with the predominance of A-lines on the contralateral side showed 100% specificity for pneumonia.[43] However, even when associated with artifacts signifying a possible concomitant consolidation their sensitivity is only as high as 14%.[43] Dynamic air bronchograms, defined as linear hyperechoic artifacts within the consolidation with greater than 1 mm centrifugal movement with inspiration, help to differentiate pneumonia from atelectasis.[48] The presence of bilateral B-lines defines the alveolar-interstitial syndrome: a collection of disease processes encompassing pulmonary edema, ARDS, noncardiogenic pulmonary edema (Boxes 6–8, Fig. 15), and diffuse interstitial lung disease.[49] Bilateral anterior B-lines showed a sensitivity of 97% and a specificity of 95% as well as a PPV of 87% and NPV of 99% for the diagnosis of CHF.[43] The resolution of B-lines may also be used to monitor therapy.[46] Lung findings in patients with COPD distinguish

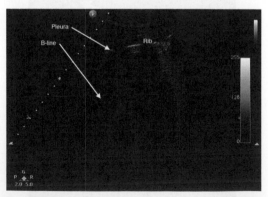

Fig. 14. B-lines. The hyperechoic line near the footprint of the image represents the pleural line. The rib interrupts this line and produces a distal shadow. Multiple hyperechoic reverberation artifacts can be seen originating from the pleural line, extending to the far field of the image, representing B-lines. Multiple bilateral B-lines are consistent with pulmonary edema.

Box 6
Case 2

- Clinical History

   o A 52-year-old man with past medical history of COPD, CHF, CAD, and gout complained of progressive dyspnea and increased sputum for 3 days. He was tachypneic and mildly tachycardic. He had chronic bilateral lower extremity edema, bibasilar rales, and a slight expiratory wheeze.

- Findings

   o The RADiUS examination revealed the following information: parasternal long view showed severely reduced left ventricular function; apical 4-chamber showed dilated left ventricle; the IVC was plethoric with minimal respiratory variation; bilateral small pulmonary effusions were also noted along with diffuse bilateral B-lines (see Fig. 15).

- Diagnosis

   o The RADiUS examination confirmed pulmonary edema caused by an acute exacerbation of heart failure. Successful treatment with preload and afterload reduction resulted in improvement of rales, wheezing, and oxygen saturation.

Box 7
Case 4

- Clinical History
  - A 28-year-old G2P2 postpartum female presents with shortness of breath, right sided pleuritic chest pain, mild bilateral lower extremity edema, and a productive cough with blood streaked sputum after recent vaginal delivery. The differential diagnosis includes peripartum caridomyopathy, hemodynamically significant pulmonary embolism, and hospital-acquired pneumonia with sepsis.

- Findings
  - The RADiUS exam reveals the following information: parasternal long view shows no reduction in left ventricular function. The apical four-chamber view shows normal right ventricular size. Examination of the IVC shows greater than 50% collapse with spontaneous respiration (see **Fig. 18**). Ultrasound of the pleura shows B lines in the right anterior lung fields (see **Fig. 14**) and A lines on the left (see **Fig. 10**).

- Diagnosis
  - Based on the RADiUS exam this patient most likely has pneumonia with sepsis and requires initiation of early goal directed therapy with fluids and antibiotics.

Box 8
Case 5

- Clinical History
  - A 38-year-old business executive was brought directly from the airport to the local emergency department in Florida after a 5-day skiing vacation in Colorado, complaining of dyspnea on exertion. In addition he complained of nonproductive cough, fatigue, nausea, headache, and bilateral lower extremity muscle cramps. Family history was significant for thromboembolism. The physical examination showed decreased breath sounds bilaterally, tachypnea, tachycardia, bilateral positive Homans sign, and pulse oximetry of 92% on room air.

- Findings
  - The RADiUS examination revealed the following information: parasternal long and apical 4-chamber views showed normal left ventricular function. The IVC collapsed greater than 50% with spontaneous respiration. Examination of the pleura showed diffuse bilateral B-lines (see **Fig. 15**).

- Diagnosis
  - As a result of sleeping at 3657 m (12,000 ft) for 4 nights, this patient had developed high-altitude pulmonary edema. The bilateral B-lines, as well as normal cardiac and IVC views, were consistent with noncardiogenic pulmonary edema.

themselves from the disease processes mentioned earlier by a lack of diffuse B-lines.[43,50]

Research does not support sonographic assessment of the lungs or pleura for PE. A study in 2005 by Mathis and colleagues[51] used thoracic ultrasonography to search for triangular or rounded pleural-based lesions as well as unilateral pleural effusion, which may indicate pulmonary emboli. However, this single study of 352 patients had poor sensitivity. Using ultrasonography to diagnose PE has not replaced either computed tomography angiography or ventilation-perfusion scintigraphy. Ultrasound is not sufficiently sensitive to rule out PE. As noted earlier the cardiac examination may help to provide insight into the presence of a hemodynamically significant PE.

Some dyspnea protocols include lower extremity venous ultrasonography to rule out DVT. Several studies have reported that emergency physicians and other clinicians can be accurate and fast in their diagnosis of DVT.[52–55] The inclusion of a DVT evaluation significantly increases time spent performing the ultrasonographic assessment of dyspnea. This examination can be selectively added in cases of suspected PE/DVT.

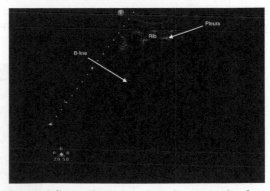

Fig. 15. B-lines. The hyperechoic line near the footprint of the image represents the pleural line. The rib interrupts this line and produces a distal shadow. Multiple hyperechoic reverberation artifacts can be seen originating from the pleural line, extending to the far field of the image, representing B-lines. Multiple bilateral B-lines are consistent with a patient with the alveolar-interstitial syndrome: CHF exacerbation, ARDS, diffuse interstitial lung disease, or noncardiogenic pulmonary edema.

- Clinical History
  - A 46-year-old man on hemodialysis complained of dyspnea and a cough after missing dialysis. He was diaphoretic, anxious, and moderately distressed, with mild crackles at the bases bilaterally, tachycardic with 3/6 systolic ejection murmur, and jugular venous distention.
- Findings
  - The RADiUS examination revealed the following information: subxiphoid and apical 4-chamber views showed pericardial effusion with right ventricular collapse during diastole; the IVC was dilated and did not collapse with respiration, and the pericardial effusion was visible (see **Fig. 16**); evaluation of the pleura showed scattered B-lines.
- Diagnosis
  - The RADiUS examination confirmed that cardiac tamponade was present with increased pressure in the pericardial effusion. There was collapse of the right ventricle in diastole and the right atrium in systole. The IVC was plethoric and did not change significantly with respiration.

Pleural Effusion

Ultrasound is an excellent tool to identify pleural effusions. These images are easy to obtain for most physicians, because they require only a modification of the hepatorenal and splenorenal views currently used for the FAST examination

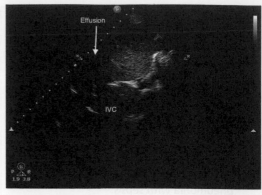

Fig. 16. IVC viewed with a phased-array probe in the sagittal plane. Notice the anechoic space between the liver and epicardium, representing a pericardial effusion.

(**Figs. 17** and **19**). Not only can the presence or absence of an effusion be identified by bedside sonography, but ultrasonography can also aid in identifying the extent of the effusion and help simplify any associated procedures.[43,56] The evaluation of pleural effusion should be interpreted within the context of the previously performed cardiac and pulmonary examination as well as the clinical presentation of the patient. Unilateral effusions are commonly associated with pneumonia, PE, aortic dissection, and traumatic hemothorax. Bilateral effusions are associated with volume overload, noncardiogenic pulmonary edema, and CHF.[43]

Ultrasound was also capable of accurately predicting the size of pleural effusions (**Box 10**; **Fig. 19**), which can be helpful when considering a thoracentesis on a mechanically ventilated

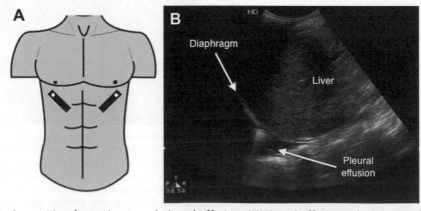

Fig. 17. (*A*) Probe position for evaluation of pleural effusion. (*B*) Pleural effusion, which is noted to be present secondary to the lack of mirror-image artifact. As seen in this image there is no mirror image artifact superior to the diaphragm. A small anechoic triangle of fluid can be seen superior to the diaphragm, suggesting a small pleural effusion.

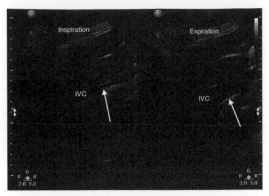

Fig. 18. Split-screen image showing collapse of the IVC during normal respiration. The arrow is directed to an area approximately 2 cm caudal to the junction of the hepatic vein and IVC. Notice that the IVC experiences almost complete collapse during normal respiration, which suggests that the patient will likely respond to the administration of fluids.

patient. Vignon and colleagues[57] showed a significant correlation between the expiratory interpleural distance at the thoracic base and the presence of significant pleural effusion. In their study a interpleural distance of more than 45 mm (right) or more than 50 mm (left) was predictive of a pleural effusion volume greater then or equal to 800 mL, with a sensitivity of 94% and 100% and a specificity of 76% and 67%, respectively. Balik and colleagues[58] conducted a study on 81 ventilator-dependent patients in an ICU and showed that the volume (mL) of pleural effusion could be accurately estimated by the formula SP (maximum distance, measured in mm, between the visceral and parietal pleura at end expiration) × 20. However, the mean prediction error for this study was 158.4 ± 160.6 mL. A more recent article by Pneumatikos and colleagues[59] suggests using

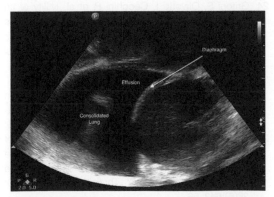

Fig. 19. Large pleural effusion viewed with the curvilinear probe in the coronal plane. Notice the large anechoic space superior to the diaphragm. When large pleural effusions are present, it is not unusual to see consolidated lung tissue floating in the effusion.

Box 10
Case 7

- Clinical History
  - A 66-year-old woman with a past medical history of COPD and right-sided breast cancer and mastectomy several years previously presented with progressive dyspnea and cough with occasional blood-streaked sputum. Her physical examination was remarkable for tachycardia, tachypnea, pulse oximetry 93% on room air, and decreased breath sounds on the right side. The EKG noted a narrow complex sinus tachycardia.
- Findings
  - The RADiUS examination revealed the following information: parasternal long and apical 4-chamber views showed normal left ventricular function; the IVC was normal in size and varied less than 50% with spontaneous respiration.
- Diagnosis
  - Examination of the right thorax revealed a large pleural effusion (see **Fig. 19**). Given the patient's clinical status, an ultrasound-guided thoracentesis was indicated.

a cutoff of more than 50 mm between the posterior chest wall and the lung on ultrasonography as highly predictive for the presence of an effusion that contains greater than 500 mL of free fluid. In these studies thoracentesis performed under ultrasonographic guidance led to a reduced complication rate.

SUMMARY

The RADiUS examination has the ability to change clinical practice by rapidly narrowing the differential diagnosis and allowing the clinician to administer definitive therapy. This real-time bedside sonographic examination combines research from cardiology, radiology, critical care, and emergency medicine. Although its ability to diagnose some important conditions such as PE may be limited, the RADiUS examination is specific for multiple disease processes. Future research may show that the outcomes and lengths of stay of patients can be improved by this focused examination.

REFERENCES

1. Rozycki GS, Ochsner MG, Schmidt JA, et al. A prospective study of surgeon-performed ultrasound as the primary adjuvant modality for injured

patient assessment. J Trauma 1995;39(3):492–8 [discussion: 498–500].

2. Jones AE, Tayal VS, Sullivan DM, et al. Randomized, controlled trial of immediate versus delayed goal-directed ultrasound to identify the cause of nontraumatic hypotension in emergency department patients. Crit Care Med 2004;32(8):1703–8.

3. Perera P, Mailhot T, Riley D, et al. The RUSH exam: Rapid Ultrasound in SHock in the evaluation of the critically ill. Emerg Med Clin North Am 2010;28(1): 29–56, vii.

4. Kirkpatrick AW, Sirois M, Laupland KB, et al. Hand-held thoracic sonography for detecting post-traumatic pneumothoraces: the Extended Focused Assessment with Sonography for Trauma (EFAST). J Trauma 2004;57(2):288–95.

5. Moore CL, Molina AA, Lin H. Ultrasonography in community emergency departments in the United States: access to ultrasonography performed by consultants and status of emergency physician-performed ultrasonography. Ann Emerg Med 2006; 47(2):147–53.

6. Moore CL, Gregg S, Lambert M. Performance, training, quality assurance, and reimbursement of emergency physician-performed ultrasonography at academic medical centers. J Ultrasound Med 2004;23(4):459–66.

7. Jones A, Tayal V, Kline J. Focused training of emergency medicine residents in goal-directed echocardiography: a prospective study. Acad Emerg Med 2003;10(10):1054–8.

8. Hauser A. The emerging role of echocardiography in the emergency department. Ann Emerg Med 1989; 18(12):1298–303.

9. Kimura B, Bocchicchio M, Willis C, et al. Screening cardiac ultrasonographic examination in patients with suspected cardiac disease in the emergency department. Am Heart J 2001;142(2):324–30.

10. Labovitz AJ, Noble VE, Bierig M, et al. Focused cardiac ultrasound in the emergent setting: a consensus statement of the American Society of Echocardiography and American College of Emergency Physicians. J Am Soc Echocardiogr 2010; 23(12):1225–30.

11. Mandavia D, Hoffner R, Mahaney K, et al. Bedside echocardiography by emergency physicians. Ann Emerg Med 2001;38(4):377–82.

12. Tayal V, Kline J. Emergency echocardiography to detect pericardial effusion in patients in PEA and near-PEA states. Resuscitation 2003;59(3): 315–8.

13. Otto CM. Textbook of clinical echocardiography. China: Saunders Elsevier; 2009. p. 608.

14. Blaivas M. Incidence of pericardial effusion in patients presenting to the emergency department with unexplained dyspnea. Acad Emerg Med 2001;8(12):1143–6.

15. Ameli S, Shah PK. Cardiac tamponade. Pathophysiology, diagnosis, and management. Cardiol Clin 1991;9(4):665–74.

16. Moore C, Rose G, Tayal V, et al. Determination of left ventricular function by emergency physician echocardiography of hypotensive patients. Acad Emerg Med 2002;9(3):186–93.

17. Amico AF, Lichtenberg GS, Reisner SA, et al. Superiority of visual versus computerized echocardiographic estimation of radionuclide left ventricular ejection fraction. Am Heart J 1989;118(6): 1259–65.

18. van Royen N, Jaffe CC, Krumholz HM, et al. Comparison and reproducibility of visual echocardiographic and quantitative radionuclide left ventricular ejection fractions. Am J Cardiol 1996;77(10): 843–50.

19. Randazzo MR, Snoey ER, Levitt MA, et al. Accuracy of emergency physician assessment of left ventricular ejection fraction and central venous pressure using echocardiography. Acad Emerg Med 2003; 10(9):973–7.

20. Melamed R, Sprenkle MD, Ulstad VK, et al. Assessment of left ventricular function by intensivists using hand-held echocardiography. Chest 2009;135(6): 1416–20.

21. McConnell M, Solomon S, Rayan M, et al. Regional right ventricular dysfunction detected by echocardiography in acute pulmonary embolism. Am J Cardiol 1996;78(4):469–73.

22. Bomann JS, Moore C. Emergency department echocardiogram of right ventricle thrombus and McConnell's sign in a patient with dyspnea. Acad Emerg Med 2009;16(5):474.

23. Nazeyrollas P, Metz D, Jolly D, et al. Use of transthoracic Doppler echocardiography combined with clinical and electrocardiographic data to predict acute pulmonary embolism. Eur Heart J 1996; 17(5):779–86.

24. Grifoni S, Olivotto I, Cecchini P, et al. Utility of an integrated clinical, echocardiographic, and venous ultrasonographic approach for triage of patients with suspected pulmonary embolism. Am J Cardiol 1998;82(10):1230–5.

25. Mansencal N, Vieillard-Baron A, Beauchet A, et al. Triage patients with suspected pulmonary embolism in the emergency department using a portable ultrasound device. Echocardiography 2008;25(5):451–6.

26. Wells PS, Anderson DR, Ginsberg J. Assessment of deep vein thrombosis or pulmonary embolism by the combined use of clinical model and noninvasive diagnostic tests. Semin Thromb Hemost 2000; 26(6):643–56.

27. Kline JA, Courtney DM, Kabrhel C, et al. Prospective multicenter evaluation of the pulmonary embolism rule-out criteria. J Thromb Haemost 2008;6(5): 772–80.

28. Kircher BJ, Himelman RB, Schiller NB. Noninvasive estimation of right atrial pressure from the inspiratory collapse of the inferior vena cava. Am J Cardiol 1990;66(4):493–6.

29. Lang RM, Bierig M, Devereux RB, et al. Recommendations for chamber quantification: a report from the American Society of Echocardiography's Guidelines and Standards Committee and the Chamber Quantification Writing Group, developed in conjunction with the European Association of Echocardiography, a branch of the European Society of Cardiology. J Am Soc Echocardiogr 2005;18(12): 1440–63.

30. Lyon M, Blaivas M, Brannam L. Sonographic measurement of the inferior vena cava as a marker of blood loss. Am J Emerg Med 2005;23(1):45–50.

31. Wallace DJ. Inferior vena cava percentage collapse during respiration is affected by the sampling location: ultrasound study in healthy volunteers. Acad Emerg Med 2010;17(1):96–9.

32. Blehar DJ, Dickman E, Gaspari R. Identification of congestive heart failure via respiratory variation of inferior vena cava diameter. Am J Emerg Med 2009;27(1):71–5.

33. Jang T, Aubin C, Naunheim R, et al. Ultrasonography of the internal jugular vein in patients with dyspnea without jugular venous distention on physical examination. Ann Emerg Med 2004;44(2): 160–8.

34. Thalhammer C, Aschwanden M, Odermatt A, et al. Noninvasive central venous pressure measurement by controlled compression sonography at the forearm. J Am Coll Cardiol 2007;50(16):1584–9.

35. Lichtenstein DA, Meziere G, Lascols N, et al. Ultrasound diagnosis of occult pneumothorax. Crit Care Med 2005;33(6):1231–8.

36. Wernecke K, Galanski M, Peters PE, et al. Pneumothorax: evaluation by ultrasound–preliminary results. J Thorac Imaging 1987;2(2):76–8.

37. Chan SS. Emergency bedside ultrasound to detect pneumothorax. Acad Emerg Med 2003;10(1): 91–4.

38. Lichtenstein D, Meziere G, Biderman P, et al. The "lung point": an ultrasound sign specific to pneumothorax. Intensive Care Med 2000;26(10): 1434–40.

39. Murphy M, Nagdev A, Sisson C. Lack of lung sliding on ultrasound does not always indicate a pneumothorax. Resuscitation 2008;77(2):270.

40. Blaivas M, Lyon M, Duggal S. A prospective comparison of supine chest radiography and bedside ultrasound for the diagnosis of traumatic pneumothorax. Acad Emerg Med 2005;12(9): 844–9.

41. Lichtenstein DA, Menu Y. A bedside ultrasound sign ruling out pneumothorax in the critically ill. Lung sliding. Chest 1995;108(5):1345–8.

42. Kirkpatrick AW, Ng AK, Dulchavsky SA, et al. Sonographic diagnosis of a pneumothorax inapparent on plain radiography: confirmation by computed tomography. J Trauma 2001;50(4):750–2.

43. Lichtenstein DA, Meziere GA. Relevance of lung ultrasound in the diagnosis of acute respiratory failure: the BLUE protocol. Chest 2008;134(1):117–25.

44. Bedetti G, Gargani L, Corbisiero A, et al. Evaluation of ultrasound lung comets by hand-held echocardiography. Cardiovasc Ultrasound 2006;4:34.

45. Agricola E, Bove T, Oppizzi M, et al. "Ultrasound comet-tail images": a marker of pulmonary edema: a comparative study with wedge pressure and extravascular lung water. Chest 2005;127(5):1690–5.

46. Noble VE, Murray AF, Capp R, et al. Ultrasound assessment for extravascular lung water in patients undergoing hemodialysis: time course for resolution. Chest 2009;135(6):1433–9.

47. Soldati G, Testa A, Silva FR, et al. Chest ultrasonography in lung contusion. Chest 2006;130(2):533–8.

48. Lichtenstein D, Meziere G, Seitz J. The dynamic air bronchogram. A lung ultrasound sign of alveolar consolidation ruling out atelectasis. Chest 2009; 135(6):1421–5.

49. Liteplo AS, Marill KA, Villen T, et al. Emergency thoracic ultrasound in the differentiation of the etiology of shortness of breath (ETUDES): sonographic B-lines and N-terminal pro-brain-type natriuretic peptide in diagnosing congestive heart failure. Acad Emerg Med 2009;16(3):201–10.

50. Lichtenstein D, Meziere G. A lung ultrasound sign allowing bedside distinction between pulmonary edema and COPD: the comet-tail artifact. Intensive Care Med 1998;24(12):1331–4.

51. Mathis G, Blank W, Reissig A, et al. Thoracic ultrasound for diagnosing pulmonary embolism: a prospective multicenter study of 352 patients. Chest 2005;128(3):1531–8.

52. Shiver SA, Lyon M, Blaivas M, et al. Prospective comparison of emergency physician-performed venous ultrasound and CT venography for deep venous thrombosis. Am J Emerg Med 2010;28(3): 354–8.

53. McIlrath ST, Blaivas M, Lyon M. Patient follow-up after negative lower extremity bedside ultrasound for deep venous thrombosis in the ED. Am J Emerg Med 2006;24(3):325–8.

54. Theodoro D, Blaivas M, Duggal S, et al. Real-time B-mode ultrasound in the ED saves time in the diagnosis of deep vein thrombosis (DVT). Am J Emerg Med 2004;22(3):197–200.

55. Blaivas M, Lambert MJ, Harwood RA, et al. Lower-extremity Doppler for deep venous thrombosis–can emergency physicians be accurate and fast? Acad Emerg Med 2000;7(2):120–6.

56. Tayal VS, Nicks BA, Norton HJ. Emergency ultrasound evaluation of symptomatic nontraumatic

pleural effusions. Am J Emerg Med 2006;24(7): 782–6.

57. Vignon P, Chastagner C, Berkane V, et al. Quantitative assessment of pleural effusion in critically ill patients by means of ultrasonography. Crit Care Med 2005;33(8):1757–63.

58. Balik M, Plasil P, Waldauf P, et al. Ultrasound estimation of volume of pleural fluid in mechanically ventilated patients. Intensive Care Med 2006; 32(2):318–21.

59. Pneumatikos I, Bouros D. Pleural effusions in critically ill patients. Respiration 2008;76(3):241–8.

Ultrasound-Guided Procedures in Emergency Medicine

Chris Moore, MD, RDMS, RDCS

KEYWORDS

- Ultrasound • Emergency medicine
- Ultrasound-guided procedures • Central venous access
- Emergency ultrasound • Patient safety • Medical errors

Ultrasound may be used as an adjunct in many common procedures performed in emergency medicine, and has been demonstrated to improve effectiveness and reduce complications in diverse applications. Although the evidence is strongest for ultrasound guidance in central venous access, the use of ultrasound has been studied in many areas of procedural guidance.

Emergent procedures may also be performed by consultants in a location other than the emergency department (ED). Some of these procedures may be similar or identical to procedures performed by emergency physicians (EPs) in the ED. This article focuses on procedures that are commonly performed by emergency physicians that may benefit from ultrasound guidance.

TRAINING AND CREDENTIALING FOR ULTRASOUND-GUIDED PROCEDURES

Ultrasound is a user-dependent technology and experience using ultrasound in procedures will improve success. How much experience is necessary to use ultrasound effectively is controversial, incompletely studied, and will vary among individuals. Although guidelines have often focused on numbers of examinations or procedures, emphasis has shifted in the past several years to assessing competency rather than simply counting how many examinations or procedures have been performed.

The effective use of ultrasound includes a basic understanding of the physics and instrumentation of ultrasound as well as psychomotor and cognitive elements of image acquisition and interpretation.

The American Medical Association has endorsed specialty-specific guidelines for ultrasound training.[1] Within emergency medicine, the American College of Emergency Physicians (ACEP) has provided the most comprehensive specialty-specific guidelines for the use of emergency ultrasound, first published in 2001 and revised in 2008.[2,3] ACEP describes both residency-based and practice-based approaches to training in point-of-care ultrasound. Although the 2008 guidelines place more emphasis on competency rather than numbers, ACEP has generally recommended 150 total examinations with 25 to 50 in each specific area as a minimum for competency in diagnostic ultrasound. Procedural ultrasound is included in these guidelines; however, specific numbers of procedures required for competency have not been defined.

Privileging for the use of ultrasound as an adjunct for procedural guidance is generally a function of a local hospital or group credentialing committee. In most cases, EPs will be privileged to perform a procedure without ultrasound guidance. Additional proctoring and experience performing an ultrasound-guided procedure may be helpful, but many credentialing committees do not require a specific number of documented ultrasound-guided procedures as long as general principles of ultrasound are understood and sterile procedures are followed. In some cases, privileging guidelines may include a certain number of

Department of Emergency Medicine, Yale University School of Medicine, 464 Congress Avenue, Suite 260, New Haven, CT 06519, USA
E-mail address: chris.moore@yale.edu

Ultrasound Clin 6 (2011) 277–289
doi:10.1016/j.cult.2011.03.005

proctored procedures before credentialing. Other avenues for training and assessing competency, including Web-based training and simulated procedures using phantoms have been advocated.[4,5]

GENERAL PRINCIPLES

The use of ultrasound to guide procedures generally involves directing a metallic object (usually a needle) into the correct area of interest. Although the specifics of individual procedures are discussed in more detail in the following sections, there are general principles and considerations that apply to most ultrasound-guided procedures. As with all procedures, appropriate consent should be obtained and a "time-out" performed with verification of correct side.

Machine and Transducer Selection

There are a wide variety of ultrasound scanners available, from high-performance cart-based equipment to handheld machines. Image quality in the portable and ultra-portable is improving and in most cases is adequate for procedural guidance, although improved visualization will aid in difficult procedures.

Most ultrasound-guided procedures are best performed with a high-frequency linear probe. Most procedures performed in the ED are relatively superficial and benefit from the increased resolution of high-frequency probes. In addition, the linear array allows localization of the structures of interest directly below the probe.

In situations where a structure of interest is particularly deep, a lower frequency curvilinear probe may be more appropriate, and in difficult to examine areas (peritonsillar, supraclavicular fossa) a high-frequency endocavitary probe may be most appropriate.

A specific preset for "procedural" or "vascular access" may optimize visualization of the needle. If these are not available, the best preset is usually "vascular" or "soft tissue." Tissue harmonic imaging may help to highlight the border of a fluid-filled structure.

Static and Dynamic Imaging

Ultrasound guidance for procedures can be static or dynamic. Static guidance involves assessing the area of interest and using ultrasound to note or mark where the needle should enter, at what angle, and so forth. Dynamic guidance involves watching the needle in real time, which can be done by the person performing the procedure (1-person), or by an additional person who does only the imaging while the other performs the procedure (2-person).

One-person dynamic guidance is a technique that involves simultaneous performance, ultrasound visualization, and visual monitoring of the procedure. This takes time and practice to master; however, for procedures involving small structures (especially nerve blocks and peripheral vascular access), 1-person dynamic imaging is preferred.[6]

For other procedures where there is a large amount of fluid, in particular when the transducer may actually interfere with where the needle is placed for the procedure, a static technique may be preferable. This is often the case with paracentesis, thoracentesis, and pericardiocentesis, particularly when large amounts of fluid are present.

Plane of Interrogation and Guidance

It is best to scan through the area of interest in 2 orthogonal planes to get a complete visualization of the anatomy and any pathology before any procedure. However, in a dynamic procedure the needle must be visualized in a single plane as the actual procedure is taking place. Relative to a needle, the 2 options are "in-plane" and "out-of-plane" (**Figs. 1** and **2**). Although the out-of-plane may be easier to use at first,[7] most sonologists prefer the in-plane approach for procedural guidance because the entire shaft of the needle, including the tip, is more easily visualized.[8] There are times when a short axis may have an advantage, particularly in locating the center of a small linear structure, such as a peripheral vein. In dynamic procedural guidance, the plane may be changed or adjusted during the procedure.

The other axis to be considered is long axis versus short axis relative to a tubular structure, such as a vessel, nerve, or tendon. A combination of long axis or short axis and in-plane or out-of-plane may be used. For example, an in-plane long axis approach may be preferable for central vascular access, whereas an in-plane short axis approach to a nerve may be best.

Sterile Technique

Sterile technique should be observed for most invasive procedures. This is best accomplished with a sterile probe cover kit designed for the specific probe. These kits will typically include a nonlatex cover that the probe can be lowered into as well as sterile gel for the outside of the cover. Although it is possible to use a sterile probe cover as a single operator, an assistant is very helpful. Gel should also be placed inside of the cover, but it does not need to be sterile. Although commercial probe covers are easiest to use, sterile gloves can also be accommodated to cover the probe if commercial probe covers are not available.

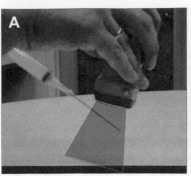
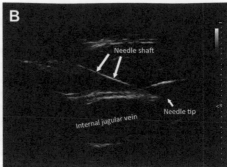

Fig. 1. In-plane visualization of needle: *A* shows how the linear probe and the plane of the ultrasound is oriented relative to the needle; *B* shows how this should appear as a needle is advanced into a vessel using the in-plane approach (and long axis of the vessel). This approach has the advantage of visualizing the entire needle shaft and tip.

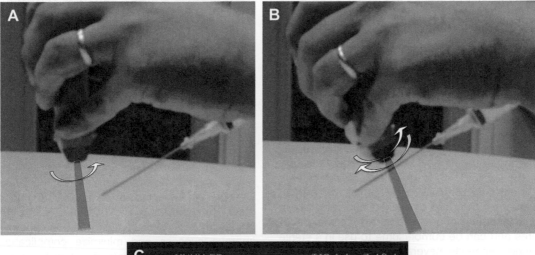

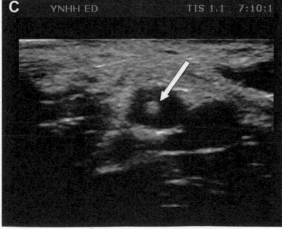

Fig. 2. Out-of-plane needle visualization: *A* and *B* show how the needle is oriented relative to the probe in an out-of-plane approach; *C* shows the "target sign" of the needle within the vessel. Although in this approach it is easier to find the vessel and the approach allows centering over the middle of the vessel, the plane of the ultrasound will need to be "fanned" (*curved arrows* in *A* and *B*) to find the tip, as a plane through the shaft will show the same image as *C*, while the tip may be deeper (*arrows*).

Certain procedures are not necessarily sterile, but should be performed in a clean manner. The probe should also be protected from blood or bodily fluids when possible by using a glove or tegaderm cover, again with gel on both the inside and the outside. The water-based gel available at the bedside for rectal examinations ("surgi-lube") is also typically sterile.

Other Equipment

Although each procedure requires the supplies that would be used for the same procedure performed without ultrasound guidance, there are a few specialized supplies that may be helpful for ultrasound guidance.

For peripheral vascular access, a longer catheter is essential for vessels deeper than a few millimeters to minimize dislodgement. Most standard intravenous (IV) catheters are 1.25 inches, with catheters of 1.88 inches and larger being more useful for ultrasound-guided peripheral access.

An echogenic needle tip with microabrasions on the bevel may aid in needle tip visualization for central venous access or other procedures. Some ultrasound scanner manufacturers are also creating presets that are better at recognizing the needle.

Needle guidance aids are improving and becoming more widely available. Traditional biopsy guides use a needle guide that is physically attached to the probe, resulting in a set trajectory for the needle that is displayed on the screen. Although these may be helpful in certain situations,[9] they are at a fixed and fairly steep angle that may not be appropriate for some procedures and can be cumbersome to use in a sterile manner. Recently, several needle-guidance techniques have become commercially available using stereotactic and magnetic positioning to anticipate the path of the needle without a physical attachment to the probe and allowing for different angles of approach. These will undoubtedly improve the ease and success of ultrasound procedures.

VASCULAR ACCESS

Vascular access is critical to emergency medicine, and ultrasound guidance of vascular access procedures can be invaluable in increasing success rates and reducing complications. Use of ultrasound guidance for central venous access procedures has been cited by the Agency for Healthcare Research and Quality as one of the top ways to reduce medical errors in the United States. For patients who do not require central access but have difficult peripheral access,

ultrasound can potentially save the patient from a more invasive procedure.

When using ultrasound for vascular access, it is critical to differentiate veins from arteries. Veins are more easily compressible than arteries and are nonpulsatile. Although this difference may be obvious for central veins in a well-hydrated patient, it may be more challenging for peripheral vessels, particularly if the patient is dehydrated or hypotensive. Although color flow Doppler (CFD) may be helpful, it is recommended that any vessel in question be partially compressed (into an oval shape) and watched for a few seconds to be sure there are no arterial pulsations. In general, veins are easily compressible, although arteries may also compress with enough pressure or in a hypotensive patient. Absence of complete compression of a vein typically indicates a thrombus.

ULTRASOUND-GUIDED CENTRAL VENOUS ACCESS

There are approximately 5 million central venous catheter (CVC) procedures performed annually in the United States.[10] CVCs are typically performed in patients who are critically ill, have difficult access, require vasoactive or multiple medications, need long-term access, or have some combination of these factors. Many central lines are placed in the ED setting, some in arrest or time-critical situations. Complications of CVCs are estimated to occur in up to 15% of line placements.[10] Complications occurring during CVC placement include arterial puncture or laceration, pneumothorax, and others. Ultrasound guidance for CVC placement has been shown to improve success and minimize complications, particularly in difficult patients or with inexperienced operators.[11] However, the use of ultrasound for CVC placement does not eliminate risk, particularly with inexperienced operators, if the tip is not completely visualized.[12,13]

Site Selection and General Considerations

The 3 major sites for CVC access are the internal jugular (IJ), subclavian (SC), and femoral veins. Ultrasound guidance is most amenable to the internal jugular site as the landmarks may not always be obvious, anatomy may be variable, and there are no bony structures that obstruct the view. Ultrasound guidance has been most well studied for IJ access, and ultrasound-guided IJ placement has been shown to be safer than blind subclavian central venous catheterization.[14] Ultrasound may be helpful for a supraclavicular approach to the subclavian vein or in accessing the axillary vein distal to the subclavian. Whereas the femoral vein is not preferred for elective central access because of higher rates of infectious and mechanical complications,[10] it may be most accessible in an arrest situation and ultrasound may be particularly helpful in this situation.

Time permitting, before sterile preparation the intended vessel should be prescanned in 2 planes to assess for abnormal anatomy, valves, scars, or thrombus. The vein should be patent and compressible. After sterile preparation, the intended area of entry should be anesthetized and may be done under ultrasound guidance to get a sense of needle orientation and depth. A small-gauge finder needle may also be used to aspirate from the vein before the larger needle.

A 1-person dynamic in-plane long axis approach is recommended for ultrasound-guided central venous access, as this will dynamically show the entire needle, minimizing complications from a misplaced tip. However, it may be helpful to begin the procedure out-of-plane in the short axis to ensure that the vein is being approached rather than the artery, and that the needle is advancing over the center of the intended vessel. When in the long axis it is important to ensure that it is the vein that is visualized rather than the artery. If there is a question, the probe should be rotated to a short axis view and compressed to ensure it is venous.

Ultrasound guidance is often used until flash is achieved, with the ultrasound then placed aside to proceed with standard placement of the guide wire and catheter. However, visualization of the guide wire may be easier than visualization of the needle, and visualization is recommended before dilation or catheter placement.[15,16] Ultrasound may help delineate a valve or other mechanical issue, allowing for successful guide wire placement or repositioning. Ultrasound may also be used following line placement to ensure central venous placement by visualizing the right heart during an IV flush. Scanning the chest for lung sliding to rule out significant pneumothorax is recommended for any subclavian, axillary, or low IJ cannulation.

Simulated training in ultrasound-guided vascular access may help to develop procedural competency and reduce errors.[17]

Internal Jugular Access

As described previously, either a static or 2-person dynamic approach may be used, but a 1-person dynamic approach is recommended (**Fig. 3**). The clinician is at the head of the bed and the patient should be in Trendelenburg with sterile cover in place. Because the clinician is at the head of the bed, the ultrasound probe indicator should be

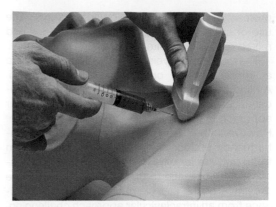

Fig. 3. Out-of-plane short axis dynamic approach on a vascular access phantom. This shows flash in the catheter on an IJ vessel being approached from a short axis. The indicator should be oriented to both the clinician's and patient's left. (*Courtesy of* Blue Phantom, www.bluephantom.com; with permission.)

oriented to both the patient's and operator's left side, so that the direction of needle movement will be consistent on the screen as it is viewed. This orientation of the indicator (to the patient's left) is opposite of most diagnostic scanning (to the patient's right).

The IJ vein is typically lateral to the carotid at the apex of the 2 heads of the sternocleidomastoid muscle, although anatomy may be variable.[18] While the patient is often positioned with the head rotated to the contralateral side, this may in fact increase overlap of the IJ over the carotid and a more neutral position of the head may be desirable if the needle can be maneuvered with the patient in this position.[19] Ultrasound should be used to identify the point where the vein is lateral to the artery and where the needle will pass through as little tissue as possible. This may include a central, anterior, or posterior approach relative to the sternocleidomastoid.[20] If the IJ is superior to the carotid, an angle of approach is recommended that will not puncture the carotid if the needle goes too deep. Higher approaches will have less chance of causing a pneumothorax.

Subclavian and Axillary Access

Before routine use of ultrasound guidance for central venous access, the subclavian vein was often the preferred site for blind CVC access based on the consistent anatomy of the subclavian vein below the clavicle. However, mechanical complications from subclavian access including pneumothorax and arterial laceration are not uncommon, and may be life threatening, as the vessel is not easily compressible and may bleed profusely into the chest before detection.[21] The use of ultrasound for subclavian access has had mixed results in the literature.

The subclavian vein may be approached via a supraclavicular or infraclavicular approach. A blind supraclavicular approach has been advocated as superior to the blind infraclavicular approach,[20] but is infrequently used in practice. However, the use of a small footprint high-frequency endocavitary probe has been shown to be feasible for ultrasound guidance of a supraclavicular approach to the subclavian vein.[22] The presence of the clavicle makes ultrasound guidance from an infraclavicular approach challenging.

Although blind axillary vein cannulation is not usually performed because of the absence of external landmarks, the axillary vein is readily visible using ultrasound. Ultrasound-guided axillary vein cannulation has been shown to be feasible with few complications.[23] The axillary vein is superficial to the axillary artery and can be found just distal to the clavicle. Because of the clavicle, it may be difficult to get an in-plane long axis view of the vessel and an out-of-plane short axis view may be required. Care should be taken to ensure the location of the needle tip during cannulation.

Femoral Access

As mentioned previously, femoral CVC access is not preferred because of increased complications, including long-term infection, but may be necessary if the torso is difficult to access such as in a trauma or arrest situation. Although blind femoral access is often considered straightforward because of the presence of a femoral artery pulse as a landmark, femoral access is associated with nearly twice the rate of arterial puncture compared with other approaches.[10] This may be even higher in situations where the femoral pulse is not easily palpable. Using ultrasound for femoral access in an arrest situation was faster and more effective and resulted in fewer arterial punctures than a blind approach.[24] This study also demonstrated that the pulse palpated during cardiopulmonary resuscitation is typically venous rather than arterial, which may make the landmark technique challenging in a code situation.

The common femoral vein is found just distal to the inguinal ligament and medial to the common femoral artery. Ultrasound can identify the saphenous vein entering the common femoral vein from the medial side of the common femoral vein. Ultrasound will also demonstrate how quickly the femoral vein will dive deep to the femoral artery as it goes distally, illustrating why a blind technique may frequently result in arterial puncture.

Hip abduction and external rotation ("frog leg" positioning) will improve femoral vein exposure and decrease overlap of the femoral artery.[25]

ULTRASOUND-GUIDED PERIPHERAL INTRAVENOUS ACCESS

Peripheral venous access in healthy nonobese adults is typically straightforward using visualization and palpation of veins. However, peripheral access may be challenging in obese or dehydrated patients, in those who have frequent access procedures (dialysis, sickle cell anemia, intravenous drug abusers), and in pediatric patients. The inability to obtain peripheral access may require more invasive measures including external jugular cannulation, CVC placement, or intraosseous access.

In difficult patients, ultrasound guidance can be among the most difficult ultrasound-guided procedures because of the small size of the vessel and vessels that may roll or be scarred down in dialysis patients, intravenous drug abusers, and patients with sickle cell anemia. It is recommended that the clinician become comfortable with ultrasound-guided IV placement in less difficult patients before attempting it in difficult patients.

The upper extremity is usually most amenable to ultrasound-guided peripheral access. A tourniquet should be used. The arm should be interrogated from mid forearm to mid upper arm to find a suitable target beginning with the antecubital fossa. If nothing is available here, the basilic vein is often a good option, on the medial side of the upper arm and not paired with an artery. The often-paired brachial veins are on either side of the artery. An ideal vein is typically about 5 mm deep. More shallow than 5 mm may not require ultrasound guidance. A vessel deeper than 10 to 15 mm becomes increasingly difficult to cannulate with more risk of catheter tip dislodgment and infiltration.

Although some peripheral vessels may be long and straight enough to cannulate using a long-axis in-plane approach, many times peripheral vessels are too small or irregular to visualize well in the long axis.

A tuberculin or insulin syringe with lidocaine may be used for patient comfort, particularly with deep IVs. A long catheter (1.88 inches or longer) should be used for anything 5 mm or deeper. In a short axis, the compressible vein should be located under the middle of the probe. The catheter should be advanced at about a 45-degree angle set back from the probe by about the depth that you are aiming for. The catheter should be advanced toward the middle of the vein with the intent of getting the tip in the center of the vessel, creating a "target sign." The endothelium of the vein may tent in some before puncture creating a target sign but not allowing the catheter to be threaded. In this case, the angle should be flattened and the catheter pushed forward slightly until a slight pop is felt and there is a flash allowing the catheter to be threaded. Backwalling may occur, requiring the needle to be drawn back slightly.

In particularly difficult patients, a modified Seldinger technique may be performed using catheters commonly used for arterial catheterization.[26] Static marking of the skin using ultrasound has not been shown to offer any advantage over dynamic guidance for peripheral IV placement.[27]

PARACENTESIS

Paracentesis is commonly performed both diagnostically and therapeutically in the ED setting, usually for ascites from liver failure. Diagnostic paracentesis is usually done to rule out spontaneous bacterial peritonitis in a patient with known or demonstrated ascites and abdominal pain, fever, or altered mental status. Therapeutic paracentesis in the ED setting is typically reserved for tense ascites with respiratory compromise.

Large-volume or known ascites may be clinically obvious and easily accessible without ultrasound. However, physical examination is insensitive and nonspecific for less obvious ascites. Ultrasound can aid in determining the presence of ascites as well as identifying the largest pocket and avoiding structures such as the inferior epigastric vessels, the bladder, and any adherent bowel. In a randomized study, the use of ultrasound was shown to dramatically increase the frequency of successful paracentesis.[28] Although ultrasound may be able to detect as little as 100 mL of ascitic fluid, it is highly sensitive once there is approximately 500 mL or more.

Depending on where the fluid collection is most evident, paracentesis may be performed in the midline through the linea alba below the umbilicus, or in either lower quadrant lateral to the rectus sheath. Although the inferior epigastric vessels should be avoided by going lateral to the rectus sheath, the use of a linear probe with Doppler may help to identify the exact location of these vessels.

With larger volumes of ascites, it is reasonable to use a static ultrasound technique to mark the point of entry on the skin and then proceed with the procedure. With smaller volumes or if there is concern about structures to be avoided, a dynamic technique may be preferable. A small-gauge needle may be used for diagnostic paracentesis, whereas a paracentesis kit is recommended for larger volumes.

THORACENTESIS

It is estimated that there are 1.5 million pleural effusions diagnosed in patients in the United States annually, and that the incidence of pneumothorax with blind thoracentesis may be as high as 20% to 39%.[29] Ultrasound is more sensitive and specific than chest radiograph for pleural effusions and may help increase success and decrease complications, particularly pneumothorax. In one series, the use of ultrasound decreased the incidence of pneumothorax to less than 2% in mechanically ventilated patients.[30]

Ultrasound has been shown to be more accurate than chest radiograph in predicting the volume of fluid that can be aspirated. A maximum measure of the fluid pocket between the thoracic wall and the collapsed lung of 20 mm correlated to an average aspirate of 380 mL, whereas 40 mm correlated to an average aspirate of 1000 mL.[31]

Aspiration of thoracic fluid should be performed from a posterior approach with the needle passing over the rib where the maximum fluid collection is present, avoiding the diaphragm and lung. A static technique is usually recommended for a large effusion, although a dynamic technique can be used (**Fig. 4**). Although large-gauge thoracostomy tubes are typically recommended when there is a hemothorax from trauma, smaller gauge catheters may often be used for simple effusions. A pigtail catheter (10–16 French gauge) is a good choice for uncomplicated effusion, particularly if ongoing drainage is desired.[32]

INCISION AND DRAINAGE OF ABSCESSES

Although abscesses may be clinically obvious, there is often a concern about whether pus will be obtained if the abscess is incised, the optimal location to incise, and the extent of the abscess pocket. Ultrasound has been shown to alter management in nearly half of cases where there is concern for cellulitis with or without abscess,[33] increasing the yield of incision and drainage of a suspected abscess.[34] Peritonsillar abscess may be particularly difficult to differentiate from peritonsillar cellulitis, and ultrasound with an endocavitary probe has been shown to assist with localization and drainage of a peritonsillar abscess cavity.[35,36]

An abscess pocket appears as an irregular hypoechoic collection underneath the skin (**Fig. 5**). It is hypoechoic but may not be completely anechoic and may show a "sloshing" motion

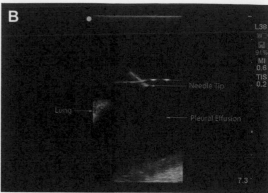

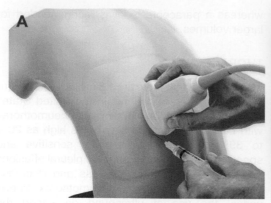

Fig. 4. In-plane dynamic thoracentesis on a phantom: *A* shows a dynamic approach with the effusion visualized using a curvilinear probe; *B* shows the ultrasound image, with the long axis of the needle entering the pleural effusion. (*Courtesy of* Blue Phantom, www.bluephantom.com; with permission.)

when pressure is applied. Recently, elastography (a color sonographic representation of tissue stiffness) has been shown to have a role in determining the extent of the abscess pocket and surrounding induration.[37]

ARTHROCENTESIS

For large effusions in large joints, such as the knee, ultrasound has not been shown to increase success compared with the landmark technique, although it did increase confidence and allow more fluid to be drained.[38] However, in smaller joints or where there is a question of intra-articular fluid, ultrasound improves identification and successful aspiration of joint fluid.[39,40] The use of ultrasound makes the emergent aspiration of deeper and more difficult joints such as the hip and ankle more feasible in the ED setting, including in pediatric patients.[41] A joint effusion

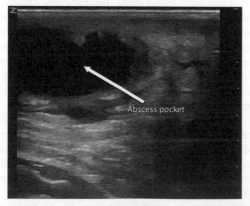

Fig. 5. Abscess pocket. This pocket is nearly completely anechoic, whereas many abscesses will show some debris. There is "cobblestoning" (a nonspecific sign of edema) in the surrounding tissue.

is identified as an anechoic space between hyperechoic shadowing bones and allows ultrasound needle localization.

PERICARDIOCENTESIS

In a stable patient, pericardiocentesis is ideally performed in a controlled situation with all available equipment, such as in the cardiac catheterization lab. However, if a patient is hemodynamically unstable with a large pericardial effusion/cardiac tamponade, emergent pericardiocentesis may be necessary. The increased availability of point-of-care ultrasound has made the possibility of detecting this entity definitively in an acutely ill patient presenting to the ED more common. Although dynamic guidance may be used, in most cases static guidance is probably preferable, as the probe is not in the way. Two approaches are described in the literature, a subxiphoid and parasternal approach. Ultrasound should be used to localize the largest pocket and shortest path to the fluid with the point of entry and angle of approach noted.[42,43] In emergent situations, a 60-mL syringe and a 2.5" or longer spinal needle may be used, although placement of a pericardial drain using a dedicated pericardiocentesis kit may be preferable for large effusions.[44]

FOREIGN BODY LOCALIZATION AND REMOVAL

Although ultrasound is not completely sensitive for detection of soft tissue foreign bodies, it may detect foreign bodies that are not seen on plain radiographs, particularly wooden splinters.[45–47] When visualized, ultrasound can be helpful in dynamic localization and removal of an object, which can be challenging when looking at 2-dimensional radiographs.[48]

NERVE BLOCKS

Regional anesthesia is useful for pain control and procedures in the ED. Simple procedures such as digital nerve blocks may be performed without ultrasound guidance, but ultrasound has expanded the range of blocks that may be effectively performed in the ED setting.[49] Ultrasound has been shown to be more effective than blind techniques with decreased complications and lower amounts of anesthetic required to achieve an effective block. Although a complete discussion of ultrasound-guided nerve blocks is outside of the scope of this article, we provide an overview of the technique and applicable blocks in the ED.

For a short-acting block, 1% to 2% lidocaine may be used. For a longer-acting block, bupivicaine may be used or mixed with lidocaine. Bupivicaine is more cardiotoxic and care should be taken to avoid intravascular injection, with some authorities recommending a lipid emulsion available as a rescue therapy. Epinephrine in the anesthetic will lower the amount of anesthetic required and will lengthen the block. Although impact of the needle bevel has been debated, most authorities recommend a short-bevel needle to minimize the chance of intraneural injection. A spinal needle may be used but care should be taken not to advance it too far.[50]

The nerve is best identified on ultrasound in short axis and will appear as a fascicular structure with a honeycomb pattern. Nerves may appear similar to tendons in cross section but have slightly larger and more hypoechoic fascicles and should not move with limb motion. With the nerve visualized in short axis, in-plane ultrasound visualization of the needle should be performed, with anesthetic deposited in a way to surround the nerve (**Fig. 6**).

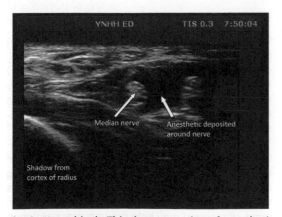

Fig. 6. Nerve block. This shows a pocket of anesthetic being deposited around the median nerve in the forearm. This nerve does not travel with a vessel. Note the honeycombed appearance of the nerve.

Upper extremity blocks that may be relevant to the ED setting include the interscalene, supraclavicular, and forearm blocks. The interscalene block is performed near the origin of the brachial plexus in the neck. The 3 trunks of the brachial plexus are identified in a "stoplight" configuration between the scalene muscles in the neck. An interscalene block provides effective anesthesia for the shoulder and upper extremity.[51,52] A significant proportion of patients undergoing interscalene block experience temporary hemidiaphragmatic paralysis, which is not usually consequential in healthy patients but makes the block contraindicated in patients with respiratory compromise.[50] A supraclavicular block is more distal than an interscalene block and does not involve the phrenic nerve but provides anesthesia for the shoulder and upper extremity. It is approached from the supraclavicular fossa, where the nerve is located lateral and superficial to the subclavian artery.[53] Ultrasound block of the distal nerves of the forearm (radial, ulnar, median nerves) has been shown to be feasible and helpful for emergency procedures.[54,55] The ulnar nerve is ulnar to the ulnar artery, and the radial nerve is radial to the radial artery, however the median nerve is not paired with an artery.

For elderly patients with hip fractures, a regional block may allow for more effective pain control with fewer side effects than parenteral analgesia.[56] Nerve block for hip fracture includes the femoral nerve block, the 3-in-1 nerve block, and the fascia iliaca block. The femoral nerve is lateral to the artery and located under the fascia iliaca, which must be penetrated to achieve a block. A 3-in-1 block is performed more laterally than a direct femoral nerve block, with pressure applied distally for several minutes to allow the anesthetic to diffuse through the fascial compartment, providing a block of the lateral femoral cutaneous and obturator nerves, which may improve anesthesia for more proximal fractures. The fascia iliaca block is performed more proximally and may perform better than other blocks for proximal hip injury or pain, as it involves the more proximal lumbar plexus. The needle is advanced under ultrasound guidance 0.5 to 1.0 cm caudal to the lateral two-thirds of the inguinal ligament, first through the fascia lata and then under the fascia iliaca where the anesthetic is deposited and should spread proximally.[57]

FRACTURE AND DISLOCATION DIAGNOSIS AND REDUCTION

Reduction of fractures or dislocations may be performed blindly or with radiologic guidance.

Although fluoroscopy has typically been the radiologic method of choice, this method involves significant ionizing radiation, and equipment may not be readily available. Ultrasound may be used to diagnose and guide reduction of long-bone fractures, with long-bone fractures of the forearm being most amenable to ultrasound-guided reduction and alignment.[58] In pediatric patients, fluoroscopy should be avoided if possible, and ultrasound has been shown to effectively help guide reduction of forearm fractures in this population.[59] Long-bone fractures will show a disruption of the hyperechoic bony cortex, and may show angulation of the 2 pieces (**Fig. 7**). Ultrasound guidance aims to provide optimal alignment of displaced fractures and is typically performed using a 2-person dynamic technique with appropriate anesthesia. A static technique (ultrasound examination after reduction) may also provide guidance.

TRANSVENOUS PACING

Emergent transvenous pacing may be lifesaving in a patient presenting with third-degree atrioventricular block. Although transcutaneous pacing may be temporarily helpful, transvenous pacing provides more definitive support. Transvenous pacing is typically performed via a centrally inserted catheter, which may be inserted using ultrasound guidance as described previously. Ultrasound may be used to track the pacing wire through the tricuspid to the apex of the right ventricle, and is helpful in determining appropriate pacer location and correcting misplacement.[60] Ultrasound may also demonstrate mechanical capture of either transcutaneous or transvenous pacing.

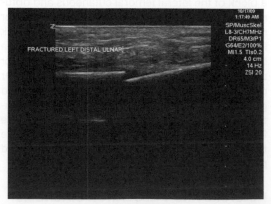

Fig. 7. Long-bone fracture with some angulation. This shows the disrupted cortex of a fractured ulna. With appropriate anesthesia, ultrasound can be used to guide alignment of the 2 fragments.

INTUBATION AND AIRWAY MANAGEMENT

Endotracheal intubation is frequently performed in the ED for definitive airway management. Although direct laryngoscopy may be possible in most patients, a subset have difficult airways. In addition to other adjunctive airway techniques, ultrasound has been shown to reliably detect tracheal as well as esophageal intubation.[61–63] The trachea is identified between the lobes of the homogeneous thyroid as a hyperechoic structure with distal scattering from encountering air. When properly performed, the endotracheal intubation will be seen as sliding just inferior to the identified trachea. Esophageal intubations will show an additional hyperechoic shadowing structure, predominantly to the left of the trachea.[64] In the case of a failed intubation, emergent cricothyrotomy may be required. Ultrasound has been shown to be of use in delineating the anatomy relevant to performing a cricothyrotomy.[65,66]

LUMBAR PUNCTURE

Ultrasound has been shown to reduce the number of failures on lumbar puncture (LP) in difficult patients.[67,68] Ultrasound has also been used to define the optimal positioning of pediatric and adult patients for LP.[69,70] Ultrasound is used to identify the gap between the spinous processes by placing the linear probe vertically and identifying the hyperechoic spinous processes with shadowing and the gap in between. In some patients, additional structures, including the ligamentum flavum and the epidural space, may be identified, helping to determine the depth of the required puncture.[71,72] The skin can then be marked in both vertical and lateral directions and the procedure performed in a static fashion.

URINARY CATHETERIZATION

Urinary catheterization is a minor but invasive procedure. Particularly in children, in whom obtaining a clean urine sample is commonly important, the use of ultrasound to ensure adequate volume before catheterization has been shown to reduce failed urinary catheterizations, especially in children younger than 2 years.[73] The use of a "urinary bladder index" (anteroposterior × transverse diameter) of greater than 2.4 cm^2 has been shown to predict successfully obtaining at least 2 mL of urine on catheterization.[74] In cases where urethral catheterization is unable to obtain urine, ultrasound may help guide suprapubic aspiration or catheter placement.[75,76] Ultrasound may also help to ensure correct placement of a Foley catheter, and may help to elucidate problems with Foley catheter function (clot, mass in the bladder).

SUMMARY

Although ensuring adequate training for this user-dependent technology is essential, ultrasound may be very helpful in successfully performing a wide variety of emergency procedures with less adverse events than a blind technique. It is an invaluable adjunct for many procedures and can be considered standard of care for central venous access.

REFERENCES

1. Ama. H-230-960 Privileging for ultrasound imaging. 2000. [cited 2011 January 19, 2011]; Available at: https://ssl3.ama-assn.org/apps/ecomm/PolicyFinder Form.pl?site=www.ama-assn.org&uri=%2fresources %2fdoc%2fPolicyFinder%2fpolicyfiles%2fHnE%2fH-230. 960.HTM. Accessed March 24, 2011.
2. American College of Emergency Physicians. American College of Emergency Physicians. ACEP emergency ultrasound guidelines-2001. Ann Emerg Med 2001;38(4):470–81.
3. ACEP Board of Directors. Emergency ultrasound guidelines. 2008. [cited 2009 February 9th, 2009]; Available at: http://www.acep.org/assets/0/16/898/ 2144/FE250562-52EF-49CD-BD93-38026154CB12. pdf. Accessed March 24, 2011.
4. Chenkin J, Lee S, Huynh T, et al. Procedures can be learned on the Web: a randomized study of ultrasound-guided vascular access training. Acad Emerg Med 2008;15(10):949–54.
5. Evans LV, Dodge KL, Shah TD, et al. Simulation training in central venous catheter insertion: improved performance in clinical practice. Acad Med 2010;85(9):1462–9.
6. Milling T, Van Amerongen R, Melville L, et al. Randomized controlled trial of single-operator vs. two-operator ultrasound guidance for internal jugular central venous cannulation. Acad Emerg Med 2006;13(3):245–7.
7. Blaivas M, Brannam L, Fernandez E. Short-axis versus long-axis approaches for teaching ultrasound-guided vascular access on a new inanimate model. Acad Emerg Med 2003;10(12):1307–11.
8. Stone MB, Moon C, Sutijono D, et al. Needle tip visualization during ultrasound-guided vascular access: short-axis vs long-axis approach. Am J Emerg Med 2010;28(3):343–7.
9. Movahed MR. Ultrasound-guided internal jugular vein cannulation. N Engl J Med 2010;363(8):796–7.
10. McGee DC, Gould MK. Preventing complications of central venous catheterization. N Engl J Med 2003; 348(12):1123–33.
11. Leung J, Duffy M, Finch A. Real-time ultrasonographically-guided internal jugular vein catheterization in the emergency department increases success rates and reduces complications: a randomized, prospective study. Ann Emerg Med 2006;48(5):540–7.
12. Theodore D, Krauss M, Kollef M, et al. Risk factors for acute adverse events during ultrasound-guided central venous cannulation in the emergency department. Acad Emerg Med 2010;17(10):1055–61.
13. Blaivas M, Adhikari S. An unseen danger: frequency of posterior vessel wall penetration by needles during attempts to place internal jugular vein central catheters using ultrasound guidance. Crit Care Med 2009;37(8):2345–9 [quiz: 2359].
14. Theodoro D, Bausano B, Lewis L, et al. A descriptive comparison of ultrasound-guided central venous cannulation of the internal jugular vein to landmark-based subclavian vein cannulation. Acad Emerg Med 2010;17(4):416–22.
15. Moak JH, Lyons MS, Wright SW, et al. Needle and guidewire visualization in ultrasound-guided internal jugular vein cannulation. Am J Emerg Med 2010. [Epub ahead of print].
16. Stone MB, Nagdev A, Murphy MC, et al. Ultrasound detection of guidewire position during central venous catheterization. Am J Emerg Med 2010; 28(1):82–4.
17. Wadman MC, Lomneth CS, Hoffman LH, et al. Assessment of a new model for femoral ultrasound-guided central venous access procedural training: a pilot study. Acad Emerg Med 2010;17(1):88–92.
18. Malcom GE 3rd, Raio CC, Poordabbagh AP, et al. Difficult central line placement due to variant internal jugular vein anatomy. J Emerg Med 2008;35(2): 189–91.
19. Wang R, Snoey ER, Clements RC, et al. Effect of head rotation on vascular anatomy of the neck: an ultrasound study. J Emerg Med 2006;31(3):283–6.
20. Mickiewicz M, Dronen SC, Younger JG. Central venous catheterization and central venous pressure monitoring. In: Hedges JR, Roberts JR, editors. Clinical procedures in emergency medicine. Philadelphia: Saunders; 2004. p. 413–46.
21. Shinzato T, Fukui M, Kooguchi K, et al. Hemorrhagic shock 3 days after catheterization from the axillary vein. J Anesth 2010;24(2):290–2.
22. Mallin M, Louis H, Madsen T. A novel technique for ultrasound-guided supraclavicular subclavian cannulation. Am J Emerg Med 2010;28(8):966–9.
23. Sharma A. Ultrasound-guided infraclavicular axillary vein cannulation for central venous access. Br J Anaesth 2004;93(2):188–92.
24. Hilty WM, Hudson PA, Levitt MA, et al. Real-time ultrasound-guided femoral vein catheterization during cardiopulmonary resuscitation. Ann Emerg Med 1997;29(3):331–6 [discussion: 337].

25. Werner SL, Jones RA, Emerman CL. Effect of hip abduction and external rotation on femoral vein exposure for possible cannulation. J Emerg Med 2008;35(1):73–5.

26. Mahler SA, Wang H, Lester C, et al. Ultrasound-guided peripheral intravenous access in the emergency department using a modified Seldinger technique. J Emerg Med 2010;39(3):325–9.

27. Resnick JR, Cydulka RK, Donato J, et al. Success of ultrasound-guided peripheral intravenous access with skin marking. Acad Emerg Med 2008;15(8):723–30.

28. Nazeer SR, Dewbre H, Miller AH. Ultrasound-assisted paracentesis performed by emergency physicians vs the traditional technique: a prospective, randomized study. Am J Emerg Med 2005;23(3):363–7.

29. Feller-Kopman D. Ultrasound-guided thoracentesis. Chest 2006;129(6):1709–14.

30. Mayo PH, Goltz HR, Tafreshi M, et al. Safety of ultrasound-guided thoracentesis in patients receiving mechanical ventilation. Chest 2004;125(3):1059–62.

31. Eibenberger KL, Dock WI, Ammann ME, et al. Quantification of pleural effusions: sonography versus radiography. Radiology 1994;191(3):681–4.

32. Liu YH, Lin YC, Liang SJ, et al. Ultrasound-guided pigtail catheters for drainage of various pleural diseases. Am J Emerg Med 2010;28(8):915–21.

33. Tayal VS, Hasan N, Norton HJ, et al. The effect of soft-tissue ultrasound on the management of cellulitis in the emergency department. Acad Emerg Med 2006;13(4):384–8.

34. Ramirez-Schrempp D, Dorfman DH, Baker WE, et al. Ultrasound soft-tissue applications in the pediatric emergency department: to drain or not to drain? Pediatr Emerg Care 2009;25(1):44–8.

35. Lyon M, Blaivas M. Intraoral ultrasound in the diagnosis and treatment of suspected peritonsillar abscess in the emergency department. Acad Emerg Med 2005;12(1):85–8.

36. Blaivas M, Theodoro D, Duggal S. Ultrasound-guided drainage of peritonsillar abscess by the emergency physician. Am J Emerg Med 2003;21(2):155–8.

37. Gaspari R, Blehar D, Mendoza M, et al. Use of ultrasound elastography for skin and subcutaneous abscesses. J Ultrasound Med 2009;28(7):855–60.

38. Wiler JL, Constantino TG, Filippone L, et al. Comparison of ultrasound-guided and standard landmark techniques for knee arthrocentesis. J Emerg Med 2010;39(1):76–82.

39. Adhikari S, Blaivas M. Utility of bedside sonography to distinguish soft tissue abnormalities from joint effusions in the emergency department. J Ultrasound Med 2010;29(4):519–26.

40. Punzi L, Oliviero F. Arthrocentesis and synovial fluid analysis in clinical practice: value of sonography in difficult cases. Ann N Y Acad Sci 2009;1154:152–8.

41. Roy S, Dewitz A, Paul I. Ultrasound-assisted ankle arthrocentesis. Am J Emerg Med 1999;17(3):300–1.

42. Silvestry FE, Kerber RE, Brook MM, et al. Echocardiography-guided interventions. J Am Soc Echocardiogr 2009;22(3):213–31 [quiz: 316–7].

43. Tsang TS, Seward J. Pericardiocentesis under echocardiographic guidance [letter]. Eur J Echocardiogr 2001;2:68–9.

44. Tsang TS, Seward JB, Barnes ME, et al. Outcomes of primary and secondary treatment of pericardial effusion in patients with malignancy. Mayo Clin Proc 2000;75(3):248–53.

45. Orlinsky M, Knittel P, Feit T, et al. The comparative accuracy of radiolucent foreign body detection using ultrasonography. Am J Emerg Med 2000;18(4):401–3.

46. Lammers RL. Soft tissue foreign bodies. Ann Emerg Med 1988;17(12):1336–47.

47. Graham DD Jr. Ultrasound in the emergency department: detection of wooden foreign bodies in the soft tissues. J Emerg Med 2002;22(1):75–9.

48. McArthur T, Abell BA, Levsky ME. A procedure for soft tissue foreign body removal under real-time ultrasound guidance. Mil Med 2007;172(8):858–9.

49. Bhoi S, Chandra A, Galwankar S. Ultrasound-guided nerve blocks in the emergency department. J Emerg Trauma Shock 2010;3(1):82–8.

50. Howell SM, Serafini ME. Ultrasound-guided interscalene block: more than meets the eye. Am J Emerg Med 2008;26(5):627–8 [author reply: 628–9].

51. Graf D. Ultrasound-guided interscalene block for shoulder dislocation reduction in the ED. Am J Emerg Med 2008;26(9):1061.

52. Blaivas M, Lyon M. Ultrasound-guided interscalene block for shoulder dislocation reduction in the ED. Am J Emerg Med 2006;24(3):293–6.

53. Stone MB, Price DD, Wang R. Ultrasound-guided supraclavicular block for the treatment of upper extremity fractures, dislocations, and abscesses in the ED. Am J Emerg Med 2007;25(4):472–5.

54. Liebmann O, Price D, Mills C, et al. Feasibility of forearm ultrasonography-guided nerve blocks of the radial, ulnar, and median nerves for hand procedures in the emergency department. Ann Emerg Med 2006;48(5):558–62.

55. Stone MB, Muresanu M. Ultrasound-guided ulnar nerve block in the management of digital abscess and hand cellulitis. Acad Emerg Med 2010;17(1):E3–4.

56. Beaudoin FL, Nagdev A, Merchant RC, et al. Ultrasound-guided femoral nerve blocks in elderly patients with hip fractures. Am J Emerg Med 2010;28(1):76–81.

57. Dolan J, Williams A, Murney E, et al. Ultrasound guided fascia iliaca block: a comparison with the loss of resistance technique. Reg Anesth Pain Med 2008;33(6):526–31.

58. Ang SH, Lee SW, Lam KY. Ultrasound-guided reduction of distal radius fractures. Am J Emerg Med 2010;28(9):1002–8.

59. Chen L, Kim Y, Moore CL. Diagnosis and guided reduction of forearm fractures in children using bedside ultrasound. Pediatr Emerg Care 2007;23(8):528–31.

60. Aguilera PA, Durham BA, Riley DA. Emergency transvenous cardiac pacing placement using ultrasound guidance. Ann Emerg Med 2000;36(3):224–7.

61. Galicinao J, Bush AJ, Godambe SA. Use of bedside ultrasonography for endotracheal tube placement in pediatric patients: a feasibility study. Pediatrics 2007;120(6):1297–303.

62. Milling TJ, Jones M, Khan T, et al. Transtracheal 2-d ultrasound for identification of esophageal intubation. J Emerg Med 2007;32(4):409–14.

63. Drescher MJ, Conard FU, Schamban NE. Identification and description of esophageal intubation using ultrasound. Acad Emerg Med 2000;7(6):722–5.

64. Werner SL, Smith CE, Goldstein JR, et al. Pilot study to evaluate the accuracy of ultrasonography in confirming endotracheal tube placement. Ann Emerg Med 2007;49(1):75–80.

65. Nicholls SE, Sweeney TW, Ferre RM, et al. Bedside sonography by emergency physicians for the rapid identification of landmarks relevant to cricothyrotomy. Am J Emerg Med 2008;26(8):852–6.

66. Orr JA, Stephens RS, Mitchell VM. Ultrasound-guided localisation of the trachea. Anaesthesia 2007;62(9):972–3.

67. Nomura JT, Leech SJ, Shenbagamurthi S, et al. A randomized controlled trial of ultrasound-assisted lumbar puncture. J Ultrasound Med 2007;26(10):1341–8.

68. Cummings T, Jones JS. Towards evidence based emergency medicine: best BETs from the Manchester Royal Infirmary. Use of ultrasonography for lumbar puncture. Emerg Med J 2007;24(7):492–3.

69. Abo A, Chen L, Johnston P, et al. Positioning for lumbar puncture in children evaluated by bedside ultrasound. Pediatrics 2010;125(5):e1149–53.

70. Sandoval M, Shestak W, Sturmann K, et al. Optimal patient position for lumbar puncture, measured by ultrasonography. Emerg Radiol 2004;10(4):179–81.

71. Ferre RM, Sweeney TW. Emergency physicians can easily obtain ultrasound images of anatomical landmarks relevant to lumbar puncture. Am J Emerg Med 2007;25(3):291–6.

72. Ferre RM, Sweeney TW, Strout TD. Ultrasound identification of landmarks preceding lumbar puncture: a pilot study. Emerg Med J 2009;26(4):276–7.

73. Chen L, Hsiao AL, Moore CL, et al. Utility of bedside bladder ultrasound before urethral catheterization in young children. Pediatrics 2005;115(1):108–11.

74. Milling TJ Jr, Van Amerongen R, Melville L, et al. Use of ultrasonography to identify infants for whom urinary catheterization will be unsuccessful because of insufficient urine volume: validation of the urinary bladder index. Ann Emerg Med 2005;45(5):510–3.

75. Gochman RF, Karasic RB, Heller MB. Use of portable ultrasound to assist urine collection by suprapubic aspiration. Ann Emerg Med 1991;20(6):631–5.

76. Aguilera PA, Choi T, Durham BA. Ultrasound-guided suprapubic cystostomy catheter placement in the emergency department. J Emerg Med 2004;26(3):319–21.

Index

Note: Page numbers of article titles are in **boldface** type.

Printed and bound by CPI Group (UK) Ltd, Croydon, CR0 4YY

03/10/2024

01040346-0013